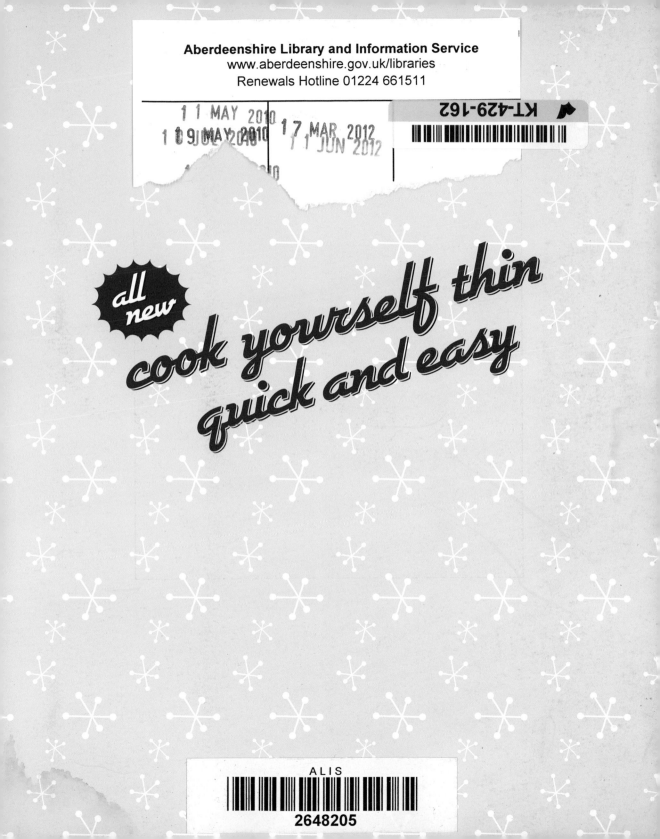

all new

cook yourself thin

quick and easy

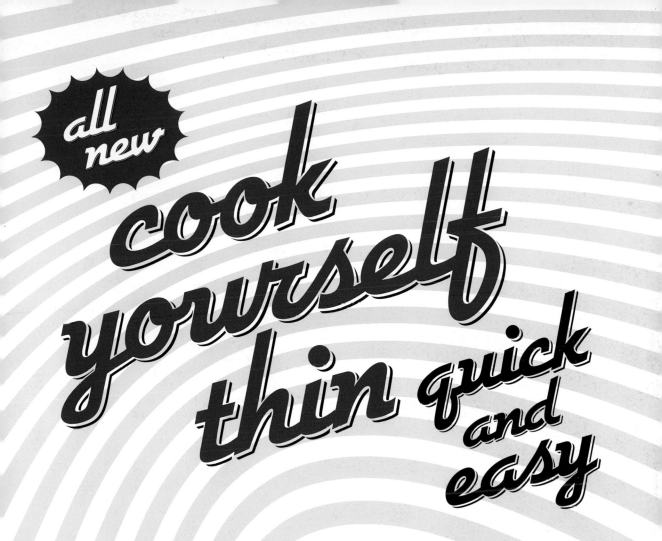

all new

cook yourself thin
quick and easy

Shift the bulge and still indulge
with over 100 new recipes

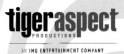

tiger aspect
PRODUCTIONS
AN IMG ENTERTAINMENT COMPANY

MICHAEL JOSEPH
an imprint of PENGUIN BOOKS

MICHAEL JOSEPH

Published by the Penguin Group
Penguin Books Ltd, 80 Strand, London WC2R 0RL, England
Penguin Group (USA) Inc., 375 Hudson Street, New York, New York 10014, USA
Penguin Group (Canada), 90 Eglinton Avenue East, Suite 700, Toronto, Ontario, Canada M4P 2Y3
(a division of Pearson Penguin Canada Inc.)
Penguin Ireland, 25 St Stephen's Green, Dublin 2, Ireland (a division of Penguin Books Ltd)
Penguin Group (Australia), 250 Camberwell Road, Camberwell, Victoria 3124, Australia
(a division of Pearson Australia Group Pty Ltd)
Penguin Books India Pvt Ltd, 11 Community Centre, Panchsheel Park, New Delhi 110 017, India
Penguin Group (NZ), 67 Apollo Drive, Rosedale, North Shore 0632, New Zealand
(a division of Pearson New Zealand Ltd)
Penguin Books (South Africa) (Pty) Ltd, 24 Sturdee Avenue, Rosebank, Johannesburg 2196, South Africa
Penguin Books Ltd, Registered Offices: 80 Strand, London WC2R 0RL, England

www.penguin.com

First published 2009

Editor: Kay Halsey
Nutritionist: Lynne Garton
Home economist: Trish Davies
Recipe writer: Kay Plunkett-Hogge
Photography: Lis Parsons
Food stylist: Lisa Harrison
Design and typesetting: Smith & Gilmour, London
Calligraphy: Peter Horridge

Printed by Printer Trento, srl

ISBN: 978–0–718–15481–3

www.greenpenguin.co.uk

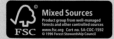

Contents

Introduction 6
Menus 16
Success stories 26

Breakfasts 32
Lunchboxes 48
Soups 70
Chicken, chicken, chicken 88
Feed me! 108
Fish 138
Vegetarian 160
Desserts 186
Drinks 204

Index 219
Acknowledgements 223

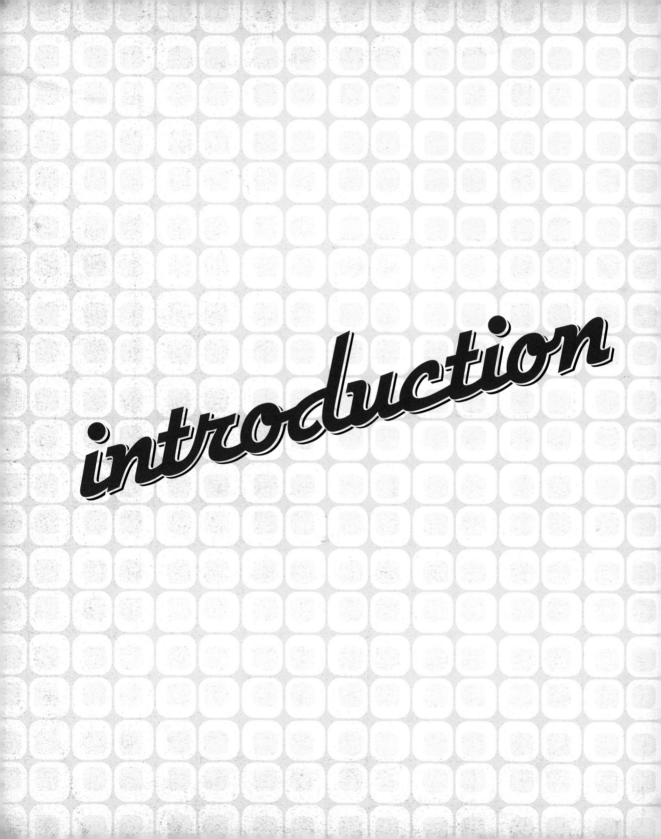

introduction

This is not a diet book. Diet books tell you what *not* to eat. This is a book about cooking, eating and simply enjoying food, and is here to tell you what you *can* eat. Simply by becoming calorie-aware, you can start to lose weight from the moment you begin. By cooking our delicious, quick and easy recipes, and following the meal plans, you'll see how tasty healthy food can be.

It's certainly not all salads. Make a few clever changes to the way you cook and the ingredients you use, and you'll soon be able to whip up a chicken curry, spicy hamburger or chocolate crispy cakes that will have you throwing those take-away numbers straight in the bin.

What's it all about?

Eating is one of life's greatest pleasures – and don't we know it! But often, when we start thinking about trying to lose weight, we believe we have to deny ourselves anything that isn't a green vegetable and give up all our favourite foods (wave goodbye to chocolate). We make eating and life in general a misery until we inevitably give in to temptation, and then give it all up.

Fortunately, this doesn't have to be the case. If you want to drop a jeans size for good, you just need to become calorie-aware. The key to weight-loss success isn't a magic potion, or only eating six raisins a day. It's simply knowing how many calories are in the foods you're eating, and how many calories your body needs. In this book we've done the maths for you, with two weeks of menu plans, and calorie counts for every recipe. Our tips and ideas will show you clever ways to cut 500 calories a day, and start losing 1lb a week. And if that sounds too difficult, you can take inspiration from the fact that half the recipes were winning entries in our competition at **www.cookyourselfthin.co.uk** to find the best healthy food, all cooked by real people in their own kitchens.

This is not a diet manual or a nutritional guide. It's a cookbook. We really believe that if you want to lose weight for good, the only way is to cook yourself to your goal. After all, if you're the one doing the cooking, you're going to be in control: you'll be mixing great ingredients together in the pan, not pouring in extra fat, sugar or salt to perk up the flavour. And when you're the chef, you can also make sure you cook clever. None of us wants to follow a diet that tells us we can't even look at a piece of bread. You really can eat what you want – you've just got to be smart about it. Love cheese on your lasagne? Then look for a really strong Cheddar, and you won't need to use as much. Want to have a full English breakfast at the weekend? Put away your frying pan, and turn on the oven. *Cook Yourself Thin: Quick and Easy* is all about showing you how small changes in the way you cook, and the ingredients you cook with, can really help you cut the calories.

What about the 'quick and easy' bit? If cooking is going to be a regular part of your life, then you need to make sure that it never becomes a chore. Recipes that are delicious to eat, but can be fitted into a busy life of work, family and friends are essential. To help, we've even picked out recipes that are ultra-quick for those of you who like to be in and out of the kitchen in less than 15 minutes – just look for the lightning bolt!

Now for the science

The most important thing to remember is that the only way to lose weight is to eat fewer calories than you use up. Once you are consuming fewer calories than your body uses, you will start to lose weight.

A calorie (or kilocalorie; they're the same thing) is a unit of measurement that tells you how much energy is in food. We need that energy to breathe and for our body to function, as well as to walk and to exercise, but if we eat more calories than we use up, then we store that energy as extra weight.

One pound of fat contains approximately 3,500 calories. So in order to lose 1lb of fat a week, you need to reduce your calorie intake by around 3,500 calories a week. On a daily basis, this means cutting down by 500 calories. To lose 2lb a week, you would need to reduce your intake by 1,000 calories a day.

Depending on your current intake, most women will lose weight at a healthy rate of 1lb–2lb a week on a calorie intake of 1,500 calories per day (for men, it should be 1,800 calories per day).

If you increase your activity, you'll burn calories that way and you may well lose more weight.

The plan

Right – let's get down to business and work out how we're going to get rid of those 500 calories a day. Five hundred may sound a lot, but just one mid-morning croissant with butter and jam and one latte will take you over that amount, so cutting down might not be quite as hard as you think. Ditch that Indian take-away you have every Friday, and you'll be waving goodbye to as much as another 1,000 calories just like that.

To start things off, we've prepared meal plans for you to follow. And for each meal, we've calculated a good calorie amount to aim for:

Breakfast: 300 calories
Light meals and lunches: 400 calories
Main meal: 500 calories
Treats or desserts: up to 200 calories a day (you can take this as 2 × 100-calorie snacks, or 1 × 200-calorie pudding)
Teas and coffee: we've included a daily allowance of 200ml semi-skimmed milk for use in hot drinks

This brings your daily calorie intake to 1,500 calories.

All the recipes in the book fit within these guidelines, and the menu plans offer lots of extra ideas for keeping to these allowances. And that's all there is to the plan. Keep to these calorie amounts and you'll lose weight. It's as simple as that.

Keeping food diaries while you're losing weight is a really great way to stay on track with your plan.

How are we going to do it?

Forget crash dieting. Those diets don't work. You might lose weight to begin with, but then, when the diet becomes too much, you go back to your old eating habits and the weight comes piling back on, often leaving you in a worse place than you were when you started!

Results might not be as dramatic as with crash diets, but making small, gradual alterations to what you eat will drop those calories and allow you to change your eating habits for good. The real beauty of this is that slow, steady weight loss is more likely to be permanent.

The best way to really see where changes can be made is to analyse what you're eating currently by writing down everything you eat (and I mean *everything* – the devil's in the detail here) in a food diary. Being as truthful as you can is key. After a week, sit down and try to see if any patterns emerge. If you notice that you're always grabbing a mid-morning snack, perhaps your breakfast isn't hitting the spot. If you're munching crisps after work, eating dinner a bit earlier might help.

After you've analysed your own eating patterns, there are five really important changes that anyone can make:

Eat regularly

We're sure you know this one already – but don't skip breakfast! Research has shown that adults who eat breakfast are less likely to be overweight than those who skip it. Plan ahead so you eat at roughly the same time each day, because then you'll be less likely to think about food in-between meals, and less likely to resort to those high-fat and high-sugar snacks. When you know you're going to be out and about, pack a few suitable foods in your bag to help you eat at your planned times. And don't let yourself get to a crisis point. Even if you've managed not to give in to a sugar craving, when you eventually do get to eat a proper meal, you are more likely to overindulge because the craving has made you absolutely ravenous.

Watch your portion sizes

If you're an over-estimator, beware! Big portion sizes mean you may be doubling your calories. If you don't know how big a portion should be, then start by cooking some of the recipes in this book to show you what a good portion size should look like. Other top tips include slowing down a bit to give your tummy a chance to let you know when it's full – try simply serving your food on a smaller plate!

Avoid high-fat snacks

With snacks, you need to think ahead, or as soon as you're hungry, you'll find yourself reaching for a muffin at the coffee shop or a packet of crisps at the petrol station. We're recommending you have 2 × 100-calorie snacks a day, so have a go at some of our great recipes for home-made snacks and keep a supply of your favourite treats from the list below. Each one is about 100 calories:

2 plain Rich Tea biscuits
2 Jaffa Cakes
2 pieces of fruit
1 low-calorie hot chocolate drink and a plain biscuit
1 small packet of reduced-fat crisps
2 breadsticks and a tablespoon of light soft cheese
3 rice cakes
1 small packet (25g) of Twiglets
1 small pot (125g) of low-fat fruit yoghurt
1 small packet of flavoured mini rice cakes
1 small cereal bar
1 fun-size chocolate bar
1 small handful (50g) of dried apricots
1 chocolate digestive-style biscuit
1 crumpet with a small amount of reduced-sugar jam
1 small glass of wine
1 pub measure of spirits with a diet mixer drink

Note: Brands vary, so always check the nutrition labels.

Eat lots of fruit and vegetables

Fruit and vegetables are fabulous, filling foods, packed full of important nutrients. At the same time, they are usually low in calories. It's because of this that the recipes included in this book are loaded with these wonderful foods.

Other tips to get your five-a-day include:

● Keep your fruit out in a bowl, so that when you're hungry, you can just grab a piece.

● Try adding just one more variety of vegetable to everything you're making. If you're making a chicken and lettuce sandwich, slice in a tomato as well. If you're making a chicken and mushroom risotto, stir in some baby spinach at the end.

● Experiment with more exotic fruit, such as mangoes and kiwi fruit, and have these as a snack instead of sweets.

● Don't forget that dried and tinned fruit (in natural juices) also count as one of your five-a-day, as well as frozen and tinned vegetables.

Don't forget the starchy foods

This plan is not about cutting out any sort of food altogether. It's about balance: eating more of certain foods and less of others. As well as eating lots of fruit and vegetables, you should also be having plenty of starchy foods, including bread, rice, potatoes, pasta and breakfast cereals. Often, people cut these foods out when trying to lose weight in the belief that they are fattening. In fact, making sure your diet includes starches that are high in fibre (such as wholemeal bread, wholegrain breakfast cereals, brown rice and pasta) can help you feel full for longer. That mid-afternoon chocolate ritual will become a thing of the past!

Exercise

You knew we'd be mentioning this somewhere, didn't you?

The best way to think about exercise is not as a chore, but just something to build into your day. Walk to work, buy yourself a bicycle, take up swimming again – it doesn't have to be all gyms and leotards if that's what's been putting you off. If you build half an hour of moderate exercise into your daily routine, you'll start to really feel the difference – not just physically, but mentally too.

Exercise is the other side of the coin in the weight-loss formula. The calories you're eating give you the energy you need for physical activities, but if you don't do any, your body will store these extra calories as fat. The menu plans and recipes show you how to put fewer calories in – but, of course, you can also use more calories up. The best weight-loss plan of all is one where you balance the two.

Food on the go

At first, you'll probably want to stick to the menu plans and calorie-counted recipes in the book, but in the future you'll certainly need to be able to buy foods in your supermarket or local sandwich shop that can fit into the plan.

To work out if a food will fit into your meal allowances, you can use nutritional labels to your advantage to see if a food is high in calories, fat or sugar.

The key things to look for on a nutritional label are:

• A food is high in fat if it contains more than 20g of fat per 100g. It is low in fat if it contains less than 3g per 100g.

• In the case of sugar, a food that contains more than 15g per 100g is high in sugar. If it contains less than 5g per 100g, it is low.

How does this translate into calorie values that you can use in your daily menu plans? If you do need to buy ready-prepared items while you're out and about, use the following guide to make your plan work for you:

● If you're buying a ready-made sandwich or salad for a light meal or lunch, choose one with less than 350 calories, and finish your meal off with some fruit.

● If you're having a ready meal in place of a main meal, choose a complete meal (one that includes rice, potatoes or pasta) at around 450 calories per serving, and serve it with a generous helping of salad or vegetables.

● For a main course dish where you need to add potatoes, rice or pasta, choose one with around 300 calories per serving and add potatoes, rice or pasta along with your vegetables.

● When it comes to snacks, desserts or puddings, choose ones that fit into your treat allowance, which is around 200 calories a day.

Lastly, please do remember that the calorie values on these pages are not intended for anyone whose calorie requirements may be different. For example, if you are under 18 years old, breastfeeding or pregnant, you should not start a calorie-controlled diet without consulting your doctor. Furthermore, these plans are not intended to replace any advice that has been provided by a qualified health professional. If you have any medical problems, it is best to seek advice from your doctor before embarking on a calorie-controlled diet.

Good luck – and enjoy cooking yourself thin!

menus

First things first. Cook Yourself Thin is not a diet. The whole ethos of Cook Yourself Thin is that diets don't work in the long term – after all, who can stick to a rigid plan indefinitely? Instead, we all have to learn to take control of the food we put in our mouths, stay flexible and accept that our tastes change according to our moods, the seasons – even which side of the bed we got out of! Sometimes you just don't fancy a salad, and nothing but a big bowl of pasta will do. Therefore, the menu plans on these pages are only intended as a guide to get you started. Once you feel confident about cooking and interpreting nutritional info on packaging, you'll be able to make up your own plans.

How to use the menu plans

The beauty of this book is its flexibility, and the way it can fit in with your lifestyle. You can choose all your meals from our big selection of recipes knowing that they have been carefully calorie-controlled and counted, or you can incorporate just one or two into your day, perhaps along with a cereal, bought snack or lunch out.

To show you how to reach a target of 1,500 or 1,800 calories a day, we have devised two weekly meal plans. Follow the 1,500 calories plan until you reach your target weight, repeating as necessary. At this stage, if you are still continuing to lose weight and don't want to lose any more, you can move to the 1,800 calories plan. If you start to put on weight with that plan, then you might need to do a bit of tweaking by, for example, adjusting your treat allowance.

As you gain experience, you can also start to make your own menu plans. You need to keep within the calorie guides for each meal, but it's easy to go ahead and switch things around – if you find your day's food has less than 1,500 calories, make up the extra with fruit and healthy snacks. Reading the nutritional labels (see page 14) and buying a pocket calorie-counting book will help you learn how many calories are in your favourite foods.

Weekly menu plan for approximately 1,500 calories per day

Day 1

Breakfast 270 calories
2 Weetabix, 10 strawberries,
125ml semi-skimmed milk,
150ml fruit juice

Mid-morning snack 100 calories
1 fun-size bar of chocolate

Lunch 315 calories
½ carton fresh carrot and coriander soup,
1 small wholemeal roll,
1 teaspoon low-fat spread, 1 apple

Snack 75 calories
1 small banana

Evening meal 424 calories
Seared ginger and soy tuna with
vegetable noodles (page 152)

Drink 100 calories
1 small glass of red wine

Daily milk allowance 100 calories
200ml semi-skimmed milk

Daily total 1,384 calories

Day 2

Breakfast 290 calories
150g pot 0% fat Greek yoghurt, 3 level
tablespoons no added sugar muesli,
3 chopped dried apricots

Mid-morning snack 50 calories
1 apple

Lunch 437 calories
Puy lentil and coriander salad (page 65)
1 chocolate-banana sunflower muffin
(page 69)

Snack 97 calories
1 small packet (25g) Twiglets

Evening meal 500 calories
Chicken stir-fry (made using 100g raw
chicken breast and a selection of
vegetables cooked in 1 teaspoon of
sesame oil and 1 tablespoon of soy
sauce, topped with chopped coriander),
50g rice (raw weight)
Marshmallow fruit salad with frozen
vanilla yoghurt (page 196)

Daily milk allowance 100 calories
200ml semi-skimmed milk

Daily total 1,474 calories

Day 3

Breakfast 311 calories
Mo'Bay smoothie (page 37)
1 medium slice toast, 1 teaspoon
low-fat spread

Mid-morning snack 82 calories
1 guiltlessly delicious fudge brownie
(page 191)

Lunch 405 calories
1 medium jacket potato filled with
½ tin drained tuna in spring water,
2 tablespoons sweetcorn, 1 teaspoon
reduced-fat mayonnaise

Snack 100 calories
1 small pot of low-fat yoghurt

Evening meal 490 calories
3 thin slices lean roast beef, 5 boiled
new potatoes, a large portion of green
beans and carrots served with 50ml
gravy (made up using gravy granules
and water), 1 pear

Daily milk allowance 100 calories
200ml semi-skimmed milk

Daily total 1,488 calories

Day 4

Breakfast 270 calories
1 toasted bagel, 2 teaspoons low-fat
spread and Marmite

Mid-morning snack 60 calories
Small bunch of grapes

Lunch 405 calories
Ham, cheese and mushroom omelette
(made using 2 eggs; 1 tablespoon semi-
skimmed milk; 1 slice ham, chopped;
25g reduced-fat cheese, grated;
5 mushrooms, sliced; 1 spritz of oil),
1 slice wholemeal toast, 1 teaspoon
low-fat spread, small bowl of salad

Snack 57 calories
Iced cardamom coffee (page 212)

Evening meal 602 calories
Seafood lasagne (page 140)
Fruit-based ice lolly

Daily milk allowance 100 calories
200ml semi-skimmed milk

Daily total 1,494 calories

Day 5

Breakfast 286 calories
Crunchy granola (page 35), made
with the optional wheatgerm; 50g 0% fat
Greek yoghurt
1 small banana, chopped

Mid-morning snack 100 calories
1 small cereal bar

Lunch 340 calories
Club wrap (1 tortilla wrap per person)
(page 60)

Snack 100 calories
2 breadsticks, 1 tablespoon reduced-fat
soft cheese

20 menus

Evening meal 490 calories
Grilled lean lamb chop (100g raw weight), mashed potato (2 medium potatoes mashed with 1 tablespoon semi-skimmed milk), broccoli and cauliflower, 50ml gravy (made up using gravy granules and water)

Daily milk allowance 100 calories
200ml semi-skimmed milk

Daily total 1,416 calories

Day 6

Breakfast 297 calories
Roast bacon, tomatoes and mushrooms with parsley gremolata (page 42)
150ml fresh fruit juice

Mid-morning snack 50 calories
100g virtually fat-free fromage frais

Lunch 400 calories
Any 350-calorie sandwich, 1 small orange

Snack 75 calories
1 small banana

Evening meal 565 calories
Luxury cauliflower and pasta cheese bake (page 165)
Green salad with fat-free dressing
Amaretto-amaretti peaches (page 192)

Daily milk allowance 100 calories
200ml semi-skimmed milk

Daily total 1,487 calories

Day 7

Breakfast 250 calories
40g serving Sultana Bran, 125ml semi-skimmed milk, 150ml pineapple juice

Mid-morning snack 181 calories
Couscous cake (page 195)

Lunch 403 calories
Hearty vegetable and lentil soup (page 74)
1 small, brown crusty roll

Snack 85 calories
140g serving of home-made fruit salad

Evening meal 480 calories
450-calorie ready meal, bowl of salad with fat-free dressing

Daily milk allowance 100 calories
200ml semi-skimmed milk

Daily total 1,499 calories

Note: All calorie values are approximate. Brands will vary, so check the labels

Weekly menu plan for approximately 1,800 calories per day

Once you have reached your target weight and decided that you want to maintain it, this plan is for you. If you are continuing to lose weight on 1,800 calories, then you may want to increase your calorie intake a little. If you find you are starting to gain weight on this intake, then you may need to reduce it slightly.

Although your calorie allowance has been increased, it is still important to keep your diet balanced. To do this, use your additional calories to include more starchy foods, fruit and vegetables in your meals and snacks. To give you an idea how this can be achieved, your calories can be spread across the day like this:

Breakfast 300 calories

Lunch 500 calories

Evening meal 600 calories

Treats/desserts
1 × 200 calories or 2 × 100 calories

Additional fruit, vegetable or starchy food snack
100 calories

Milk allowance for teas and coffees 100 calories

Total 1,800 calories

Day 1

Breakfast 290 calories
1 fruit scone, 2 teaspoons reduced-fat spread, 2 teaspoons reduced-sugar jam, 1 peach, 1 handful grapes

Mid-morning snack 105 calories
Tropical fruit selection (1 slice pineapple, 1 kiwi fruit, 2 lychees, 1 slice mango)

Lunch 468 calories
Sweet potato and apple soup (page 79)
Cheese roll (1 thin slice of cheese, 1 teaspoon low-fat spread, 1 soft brown roll)
1 fun-size bar of chocolate

Snack 84 calories
1 chocolate crispy cake (page 197)

Evening meal 685 calories
2 reduced-fat pork sausages, grilled; 2 medium size potatoes, mashed with 1 tablespoon of semi-skimmed milk and 1 teaspoon of reduced-fat spread; sweetcorn, peas and 50ml gravy (made up using gravy granules and water)
¼ tin fruit cocktail in juice, 100g ready-prepared, low-fat custard

Daily milk allowance 100 calories
200ml semi-skimmed milk

Daily total 1,732 calories

22 menus

Day 2

Breakfast 280 calories
40g serving Fruit and Fibre, 125ml semi-skimmed milk, 150ml fruit-based smoothie

Mid-morning snack 40 calories
Mini snack box of raisins

Lunch 471 calories
Greek salad (page 62)
1 pitta bread
2 medium kiwi fruits and 6 lychees

Snack 95 calories
2 rice cakes, 1 tablespoon tzatziki

Evening meal 754 calories
Beany cottage pie (made with 100g lean raw beef mince, dry-fried with 1 small chopped onion and a clove of garlic; add ½ tin baked beans, 1 tablespoon tomato puree and stock made with a beef stock cube. Once thickened, top with 1 large boiled potato mashed with 1 tablespoon semi-skimmed milk and 1 teaspoon low-fat spread, green beans and carrots
Light strawberry sponge (page 202)

Daily milk allowance 100 calories
200ml semi-skimmed milk

Daily total 1,740 calories

Day 3

Breakfast 295 calories
Grilled tomatoes and mushrooms on toast (2 slices wholemeal toast, 2 teaspoons low-fat spread, 4 medium tomatoes and 8 large mushrooms, grilled)

Mid-morning snack 201 calories
1 slice banana loaf (page 188)

Lunch 465 calories
Cream cheese, cucumber and ham wrap (1 soft tortilla wrap, 1 tablespoon low-fat cream cheese, 2 slices chopped ham, diced cucumber), 1 slice fruited malt bread, 1 teaspoon low-fat spread, 150ml orange juice

Snack 70 calories
1 slice melon topped with raspberries

Evening meal 671 calories
Garden-fresh quiche (page 162)
8 small new potatoes and a sliced tomato salad
Baked apple filled with ½ tablespoon raisins

Daily milk allowance 100 calories
200ml semi-skimmed milk

Daily total 1,802 calories

Day 4

Breakfast 300 calories
45g porridge made up using a mixture of semi-skimmed milk and water, 1 small banana

Mid-morning snack 50 calories
1 apple

Lunch 511 calories
Tricolore jacket potato (page 170)
Small pot of fruit in jelly

Snack 100 calories
1 crumpet, reduced-sugar jam

Evening meal 760 calories
Prawn dopiaza curry (100g prawns fried in 1 teaspoon sunflower oil with 1 small onion and ¼ jar dopiaza sauce), basmati rice (50g raw weight), 1 chapatti (cooked without fat) and a bowl of salad
Eton mess (page 198)

Daily milk allowance 100 calories
200ml semi-skimmed milk

Daily total 1,821 calories

Day 5

Breakfast 267 calories
Red berry compote with yoghurt and honey (page 40)
1 small brioche roll

Mid-morning snack 80 calories
2 plain Rich Tea biscuits

Lunch 430 calories
Pasta and mixed bean salad (made from 50g raw pasta, boiled and mixed with 150g canned mixed beans, ½ pepper, 2 chopped spring onions and 1 tablespoon reduced-calorie mayonnaise.)
1 small pot of reduced-calorie chocolate mousse

Snack 240 calories
50g reduced-fat guacamole, carrot sticks, 1 piece toasted pitta bread

Evening meal 550 calories
Steam-cooked salmon with soy sauce (page 150)
Rice, boiled (50g raw weight), watercress salad, miso soup

Drink 100 calories
1 small glass of wine

Daily milk allowance 100 calories
200ml semi-skimmed milk

Daily total 1,767 calories

Day 6

Breakfast 332 calories
Kiwi, banana and lime sunshine
smoothie (page 36)
1 medium slice toast, 1 teaspoon
low-fat spread

Mid-morning snack 100 calories
1 small packet reduced-fat crisps

Lunch 493 calories
Baked goat's cheese and chicory salad
(page 178)
Rocket salad, 10cm crusty French bread,
1 teaspoon low-fat spread

Snack 120 calories
Dried fruit medley soaked overnight
in tea (3 prunes, 3 dried apricots, 1 fig)

Evening meal 680 calories
Chicken in a spicy tomato sauce (100g
cooked skinless chicken breast, ½ tin
chopped tomatoes, ½ chilli, small onion,
handful of mushrooms, ½ red pepper,
10 black olives and a splash of red wine)
served with pasta (75g raw weight)
1 scoop frozen yoghurt

Daily milk allowance 100 calories
200ml semi-skimmed milk

Daily total 1,825 calories

Day 7

Breakfast 243 calories
Coconut and banana pancakes (page 38)
with optional maple syrup
150ml orange juice

Mid-morning snack 60 calories
4 dried apricots

Lunch 500 calories
2 slices cheese on toast (2 slices
wholemeal toast, 50g reduced-fat
Cheddar cheese), 150g fruit compote,
2 tablespoons half-fat crème fraîche

Snack 195 calories
1 fruit scone, 2 teaspoons jam

Evening meal 704 calories
1 pork chop with lemon and sage
(page 122)
8 small new potatoes, large portion
of cabbage
Dark chocolate and coffee mousse
(page 200)

Daily milk allowance 100 calories
200ml semi-skimmed milk

Daily total 1,802 calories

Note: All calorie values are approximate.
Brands will vary, so check the labels.

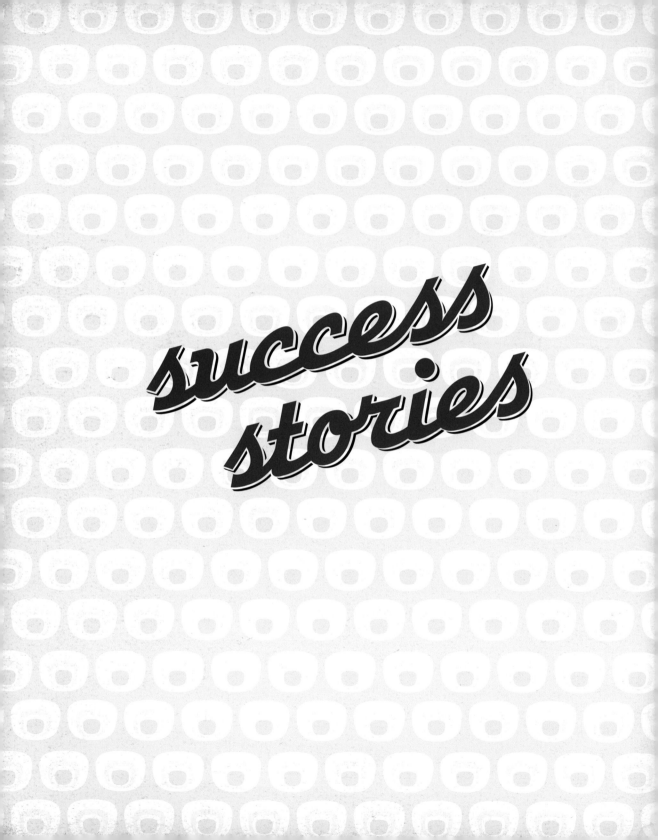

Cook Yourself Thin: Quick and Easy hasn't been dreamt up in a gadget-filled professional kitchen or written by an haute cuisine chef. It's the result of the real love of cooking and recipe-swapping that goes on in the Cook Yourself Thin community. Since **www.cookyourselfthin.co.uk** started up, our members have swapped ideas, tips and recipes. By doing so, they have motivated each other in their shared goal to lose weight. Half the recipes here came from a competition on the Cook Yourself Thin website. They also use the community to share their experiences, send encouragement and work together to follow the Cook Yourself Thin ethos. These are four success stories from people who have taken that journey.

Tamar

Tamar has a very hectic career as a fashion stylist, and decided to lose weight for her wedding. She lost 1 stone with Cook Yourself Thin before the big day, and carried on afterwards. Here, she tells us how she did it, and how the weight loss has affected her life.

Life before Cook Yourself Thin

I have always battled with my weight, but my busy job has made it even more difficult. The worst thing about being overweight for me is not feeling energetic and healthy. In a job where I am on my feet all day, I could do with the extra get-up-and-go – when I feel overweight, I'd rather stay in and veg!

What was your motivation to lose weight?

I'd just had enough of feeling sluggish, and getting engaged gave me the much-needed push to do something about it.

How did Cook Yourself Thin help?

Cook Yourself Thin has changed my whole attitude to food. I used to believe that diet food was boring, but with the website and the first cookbook, I found there are so many tasty things you can have.

What changes have you made?

Now, I always read the nutritional info on the back of packets. As well as calories, you find that some foods are packed with sugar and salt! I also measure everything; it's crucial for keeping on track. Another new thing is that I make food in advance, such as a batch of soup, so I can carry it around with me. It means I have no excuse for buying fast food.

What's the hardest thing?

The hardest thing in the beginning was monitoring portion sizes, because I was used to eating so much. Now, I sometimes have trouble finishing the Cook Yourself Thin meals!

What difference has losing weight made?

I just feel much happier, and friends have commented that I look much better, which is a great boost. I got into my first pair of size 10 jeans since I was 16 – it felt amazing, plus clothes look so much better without the 'muffin tops'!

Cherie

Cherie is 34-year-old, full-time mother to two boys aged six and two.
She has lost 2 stone with Cook Yourself Thin.

What was life like before Cook Yourself Thin?

I gained a huge amount of weight after my first son was born. I really had neither the time nor the inclination to diet, and before I knew it I was pregnant again. Well, after two years, I was running out of excuses. I never really thought I ate a vast amount, but looking back I can see where I went wrong: the wrong types of food, and portions that were way too large. I found myself going out less and less, and buying baggier and baggier clothing.

Why did you decide to start trying to lose weight?

Over the past year, I started to make a new circle of friends at my son's school, and was soon being asked to more and more social events. That was when I decided that enough was enough, and the weight needed to go so I could feel like me again. I spent hours searching the Internet for a 'diet' site to join. This is when I came across Cook Yourself Thin. At first I thought it was too good to be true! I really liked the idea of educating myself rather than depriving myself.

Why does Cook Yourself Thin work?

Cook Yourself Thin has changed the way I view food. I no longer reach for the chocolate when I'm down. I reach for the fruit and my trainers. I've found exercise really picks me up – which is not something I ever thought I'd hear myself say!

What are the most important changes you've made?

As a family, we are now eating a lot more fruit and veg. I am not afraid to venture out of my comfort zone and try new things, and I am eating better and tastier food than ever. If I want a treat, then I have one. I don't deprive myself, I just have things in moderation. My husband adores the recipes and in his own words, says he 'has never eaten so well'. I can honestly say that I haven't found following Cook Yourself Thin difficult in any way.

How has losing weight changed things?

I have lost 2 stone and I can't remember ever being this happy with myself. My confidence has grown, and my relationships with my husband and children have improved vastly. I feel that my children now have the healthy, happy mummy they deserve.

Any tips?

Drink plenty of water during the day, especially before meals!

Susan

Susan is 25, and her story is about the first ½ stone she lost with Cook Yourself Thin.

Life before Cook Yourself Thin

I've always been about a size 14, but since getting together with my boyfriend, the weight started to creep on and I went up to a size 16 – even some of those clothes were tight! I think it was due to me being content and socializing more. My weight really got me down though; and the more down I felt, the more I ate. I've never been one for snacking between meals, but I noticed I was eating a lot of rubbish and that the portion sizes were getting bigger.

What was your motivation to lose weight?

When I got engaged and we set the wedding date for a year ahead. I decided I wanted to lose some weight for the wedding. Rather than focusing on losing weight solely for that, I wanted it to be a lifetime thing. I have tried many diets, but I always seem to get bored within a few weeks. But when I saw Cook Yourself Thin on TV, it gave me the kick I needed.

Why does Cook Yourself Thin work for you?

The main benefits for me are the food diary and the online support. The recipes are great: really easy, tasty and my bloke loves them too. Since starting Cook Yourself Thin, I look at food in a different way. I have never looked at calorie content before, and it is so shocking to see the amount of calories that were in my favourite foods.

What are the best changes you've made?

When I first joined, I wasn't very experienced in the kitchen, and the cupboards, fridge and freezer were full of rubbish. When you do your first couple of Cook Yourself Thin shops, you may think it's expensive, but it does get cheaper once you have the basic ingredients in the house. I now love cooking! It was really easy to make changes to my eating habits, and I never feel like I'm missing out on anything. I did struggle to get into the habit of exercising more though.

Has losing weight made a big difference?

Even though I have only lost ½ stone so far, I feel great and I really want to continue. A few people have noticed and made comments, which are good to hear. I also felt great when I bought a dress in a size 14 again. I can't remember the last time that happened. My next goal is getting into size 14 jeans... nearly there!

30 success stories

Ejemhen

Eje is 33, and has lost over 2 stone with Cook Yourself Thin.

What were your weight ups and downs before Cook Yourself Thin?

From the time I hit puberty, I have always struggled with my weight. I have never been what would be called thin; that's fine with me, but I hated being fat. I wish I could say that there was some disaster in my life that made me put on weight, but the truth is, I put on weight because I ate the wrong things in large portions. Don't get me wrong: I was never one for cakes and chocolates. But when it came to meals, I would just eat huge portions.

Why did you decide you wanted to lose weight?

After I got married I decided that I needed to lose weight properly, because we might want to have a baby in the next couple of years. I also had all these amazing clothes in my wardrobe that I couldn't fit into.

Why did you choose Cook Yourself Thin?

I just couldn't think of what weight-loss plan to follow. I needed something that would allow me to eat what I wanted and would not force me to eat salads all the time – yuck! In the past, I had tried quite a few diets and they all worked for a while, but nothing lasted. All I can say is that Cook Yourself Thin is a godsend, and I especially like the fact that it tells me how many calories I am allowed in the day so I can lose weight.

What changes have you made?

My husband and I haven't had to make any huge differences to our cooking and shopping habits. We still have all the food we enjoyed in the past, with only minor differences. For example, if we are having Bolognese for dinner, I make sure I buy extra-lean mince, I cook the meal without oil, and I serve it without cheese on top. It is amazing how many calories you can save by doing this, and it is still a delicious meal.

What's the best thing about Cook Yourself Thin?

If I had to pick a single best thing about Cook Yourself Thin, I would say that it is the fact that nothing is forbidden. I feel like I can eat anything at all, as long as it's in moderation. People who know I'm losing weight often say, 'Are you allowed to eat that?' and the answer is always, 'Yes, I am!' I have a calorie allowance for the day, and as long as I stick to that, I can eat anything I want.

What difference has losing weight made?

The main benefits for me are that I look and feel better. When I get dressed to go out for an evening or to come into work, I know I look good, and that does wonders for my ego.

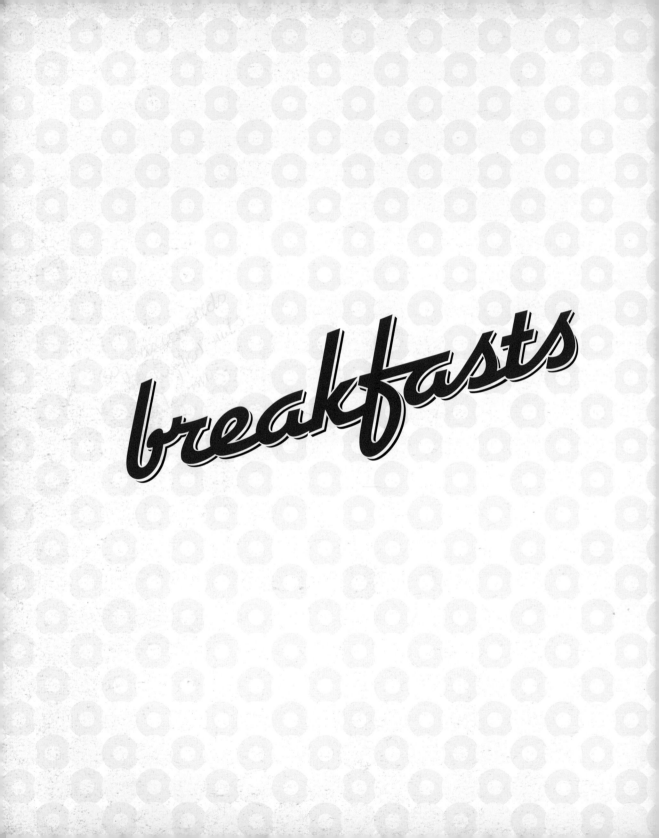

breakfasts

Start your day the Cook Yourself Thin way! Breakfast is the most important meal of the day, and should never be skipped. You might think you're saving your 300 calories for later, but the mid-morning Danish and Grande latte that you'll end up craving will set you back almost twice that. Instead, try eating some slow-acting carbs for breakfast to help keep your blood-sugar levels steady until lunch. Don't forget: girls who skip breakfast wear big knickers. It's been scientifically proven!

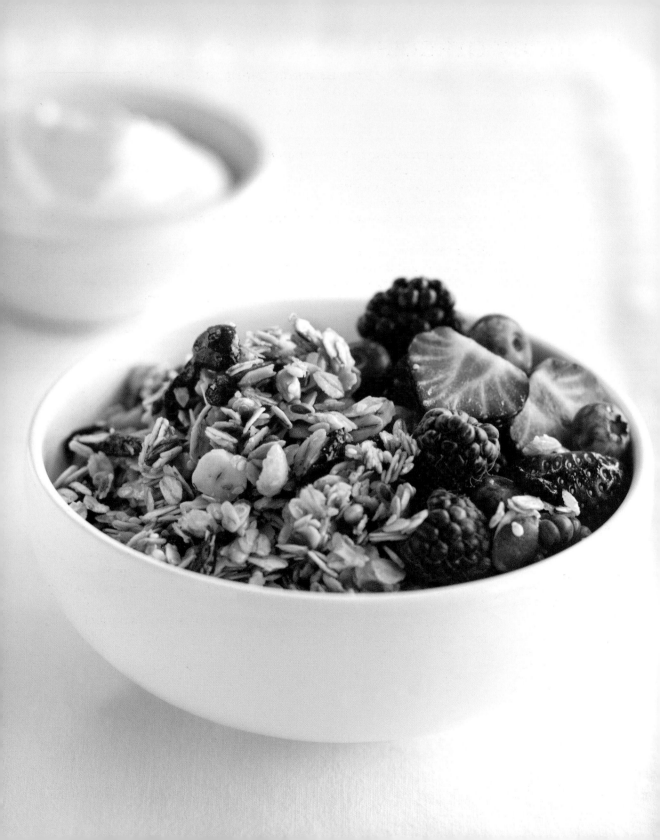

Crunchy granola

This granola is so easy to make. It takes next to no time to prepare, and it's lower in fat, added sugar and calories than most shop-bought varieties.

makes approx 450g (50g serving per person)
prep time 10 minutes
cooking time 25 minutes
183 calories per serving
185 calories per serving with optional wheatgerm

200g jumbo porridge oats
30g mixed seeds of your choice, such as linseeds, pumpkin seeds,
    sunflower seeds or sesame seeds
30g chopped nuts, such as hazelnuts, walnuts or almonds
1 tablespoon wheatgerm (optional)
1 tablespoon sunflower or safflower oil
½ teaspoon vanilla extract
100g runny honey
60g dried fruit of your choice, such as raisins, cranberries
    or chopped unsulphured apricots

Preheat the oven to 150°C/fan 130°C.
Stir together the oats, seeds, nuts and wheatgerm (if using) in a large bowl.
Mix the oil, vanilla and honey together in a jug. Add the oil to the jug first as this helps to prevent the honey sticking to the jug. Pour the honey mix over the dry ingredients and mix well so all the dry ingredients are coated.
Spread the mixture over a large, non-stick baking tray. Bake for 10 to 15 minutes, remove from the oven, add the dried fruit and stir. Bake for a further 10 minutes. Remove from the oven and leave to cool completely before storing.
This granola lasts up to a month in an airtight container. It's perfect for serving with 50g 0% fat Greek yoghurt and fresh fruit for breakfast, or even as a dessert.

tip

There are endless variations to this recipe, so don't be afraid of varying the ingredients as long as you stick to the basic ratio of wet to dry ingredients. You can take out the nuts if you want to reduce the calories. Adding 0% fat Greek yoghurt will only add an extra 26 calories per serving.

Kiwi, banana and lime sunshine smoothie

A tart, juicy smoothie full of sunny flavours.

serves 1 generously
prep time 5 minutes
222 calories per serving

120ml low-fat natural yogurt
2 kiwi fruits, peeled and chopped
1 ripe medium banana
juice of ½ lime

Freeze a few peeled bananas in plastic bags for extra-chilled smoothies, or just as a sweet iced treat. Raisins are also great in the freezer – they become chewy, like toffees.

Whiz all the ingredients in a blender and just feel the vitamin C boost!

Mo'Bay smoothie

It's smooth, Jamaican, and it sets you up for the day. You've gotta love it! Making your own smoothie is so simple, and it's really economical compared to what you pay for a bottle with a cheeky name on it in the shops. And there's a big plus – you know *exactly* what has gone into it.

serves 1
prep time 5 minutes
201 calories per serving

40ml semi-skimmed milk
75ml low-fat probiotic yogurt
1 ripe banana, peeled
100g strawberries, hulled
½ teaspoon ground allspice
1 teaspoon sliced toasted almonds

Pop the smoothic into a Thermos to take to work for breakfast on the go.

Whiz all the ingredients together in a blender.
Pour into a long chilled glass and sip. A little bit of the Caribbean at your breakfast table!

Coconut and banana pancakes

This recipe is perfect for a lazy Sunday breakfast when you want to indulge a little bit. It's so quick and easy that you won't waste any of the morning preparing it.

 serves 4
prep time 10 minutes
cooking time 3–4 minutes
193 calories per serving with maple syrup

100g plain flour
1 teaspoon baking powder
¼ teaspoon caster sugar
a pinch of salt
95ml skimmed milk
95ml low-fat coconut milk
1 medium egg
extra-virgin olive oil spray
1 medium banana, peeled and thinly sliced
2½ tablespoons maple syrup (optional)

Sift the flour and baking powder into a medium-sized mixing bowl. Add the sugar and salt.

Whisk the milk, coconut milk and egg in a measuring jug. Add the liquid to the flour and whisk thoroughly to combine. If you feel you need a slightly looser batter, then feel free to add a little water. On the other hand, if you want a stiffer batter, don't add all the milk and egg mixture. The batter should coat the back of a wooden spoon thickly.

Heat a frying pan and cook the pancakes in batches of two, three or four, depending on the size of your pan. Spritz each area of the pan you will use to cook a pancake once with olive oil.

Pour some of the batter into the hot frying pan and lay slices of the banana on top of the batter, pushing them down into the pancake. After 2 to 3 minutes, when the bottoms are nicely golden, flip the pancakes with a spatula to cook the other side. This should take less time: about 1 to 2 minutes.

Keep the cooked pancakes warm while you cook the next batch. This amount of batter should make six to eight pancakes. Serve warm with the maple syrup drizzled over.

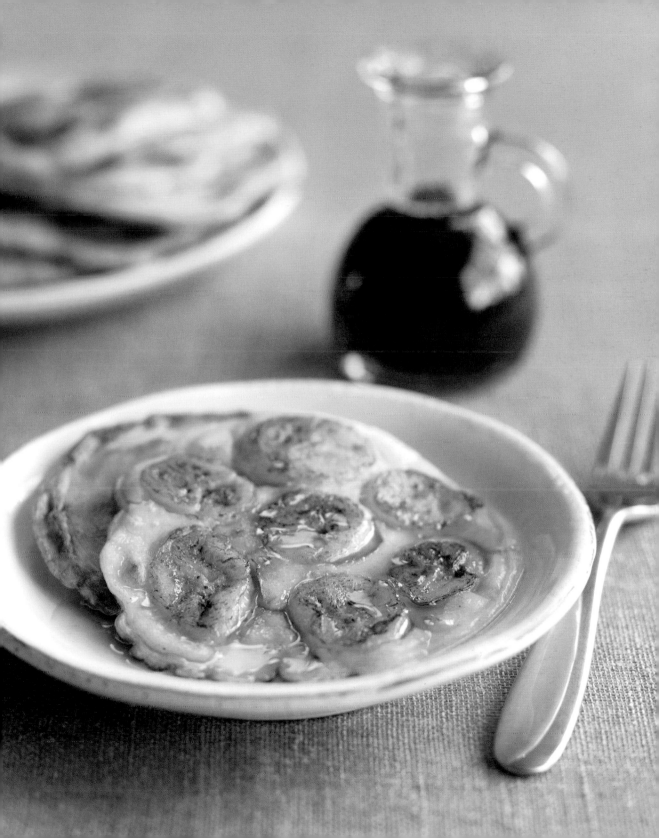

Red berry compote with yoghurt and honey

Most of the big supermarkets now do mixed boxes of red fruits (sometimes frozen) – or you can have a fun day out picking your own! This compote is also great without the honey as a light dessert.

makes 5 servings
prep time 5 minutes
cooking time 5 minutes
142 calories per serving

500g mixed red fruits (prepared raspberries, strawberries,
    blueberries, plums, peaches, redcurrants)
2 teaspoons icing sugar or sweetener
juice of 2 oranges
a dash of rose water or orange-flower water (optional)
500g low-fat natural probiotic yogurt
2 teaspoons good honey (per serving)

Wash and dry the fruits thoroughly, or defrost if frozen. Whiz them in a blender with the powdered sugar or sweetener, the orange juice and the flower water if you are using it. Put into a container and chill. Serve 100g compote with 100g yoghurt (you can even warm the compote up) and drizzle with the honey.

Make a pot of compote and keep it in the fridge for 5 to 6 days, then just grab it every morning and pour over your yoghurt for breakfast. Sieve the compote to remove any pips if you like.

Wholewheat molasses muffins

Dense, seedy, fruity – and very filling! We love the fact that these muffins are not too sweet. And they're good for you! Molasses contain iron, and omega seeds (a mixture of linseeds, sunflower, pumpkin and sesame seeds) are a good source of omega oils. They're great sprinkled onto salads and cereals as well.

makes 9 muffins
prep time 10 minutes
cooking time 20 minutes
146 calories per muffin
162 calories per muffin with optional honey and seeds

100g wholemeal flour,
   preferably stone-ground
100g plain flour
2 teaspoons ground cinnamon
   powder
a pinch of salt
½ teaspoon bicarbonate of soda
3 teaspoons baking powder
2 tablespoons blackstrap
   molasses (widely available
   in health food stores)
150ml skimmed milk
1 large egg

grated zest and juice of 1 large
   orange (or enough juice to
   make the milk up to 200ml)
1 tablespoon vegetable oil
2 tablespoons finely grated apple
2 tablespoons grated carrot
50g All Bran
1 tablespoon omega seeds
   (optional)
2 tablespoons raisins or sultanas
1 tablespoon clear honey, warmed
   slightly (optional)

The magic chemistry of baking says that you must always add the wet ingredients to the dry for muffins. The mixture must be loose, or you will end up with squashed muffins. Mix gently by hand for the lightest, fluffiest muffins. You could substitute wheat bran for the All Bran.

Preheat the oven to 200°C/fan 180°C.
Sieve both flours, the cinnamon, salt, bicarbonate of soda and baking powder into one large bowl.
In another bowl or jug, mix the molasses, milk, egg, orange juice and vegetable oil with a wooden spoon, beating all the ingredients to combine them together.
Pour the liquid mixture into the dry mixture and stir to combine loosely. Do not over-mix.
Gently stir in the apple, carrot, orange zest, raisins and sultanas and All Bran. Add the seeds, if you're using them.
Pour into a prepared muffin tin (either line the holes with paper muffin cases or lightly oil them – we think paper is easier).
Pop into the oven for 15 to 20 minutes, or until firm and fragrant.
If you want to add a little topping, drizzle the warmed honey over the top of the muffins and scatter a few more omega seeds on top.
Eat warm!

Roast bacon, tomatoes and mushrooms with parsley gremolata

Everyone loves a cooked breakfast from time to time, but all the fat in a fry-up can be very off-putting. Here's a simple solution: roast your bacon in the oven. All you need is a rack for your roasting tin so the bacon fat drips away.

serves 2
prep time 5 minutes
cooking time 15 minutes
247 calories per serving

4 rashers of lean, smoked back bacon
2 vine tomatoes, halved
2 Portobello mushrooms, wiped
extra-virgin olive oil spray
1 tablespoon flat-leaf parsley, finely chopped
Zest of 1 unwaxed lemon, finely grated
1 clove of garlic, very finely chopped
a pinch of sea salt
a pinch of freshly ground black pepper
2 slices wholemeal toast

Preheat the oven to 220°C/fan 200°C.
Place the bacon rashers on a rack in a roasting tin.
Spritz the tomatoes and mushrooms with olive oil and put them on the rack with the bacon. Make sure all your ingredients are evenly spaced out, so they've plenty of room to cook.
Roast in the oven for 15 minutes, until the bacon is crispy. About halfway through, turn the bacon and baste the tomatoes and mushrooms in the pan juices so they don't burn.
In the meantime, make the gremolata. Mix the chopped parsley, the lemon zest and the very finely chopped garlic with the sea salt and pepper in a small bowl.
Remove the roasting tin from the oven, put the bacon, tomatoes and mushrooms on a plate and sprinkle the mushrooms and tomatoes with the gremolata.
Serve with a slice of wholemeal toast.

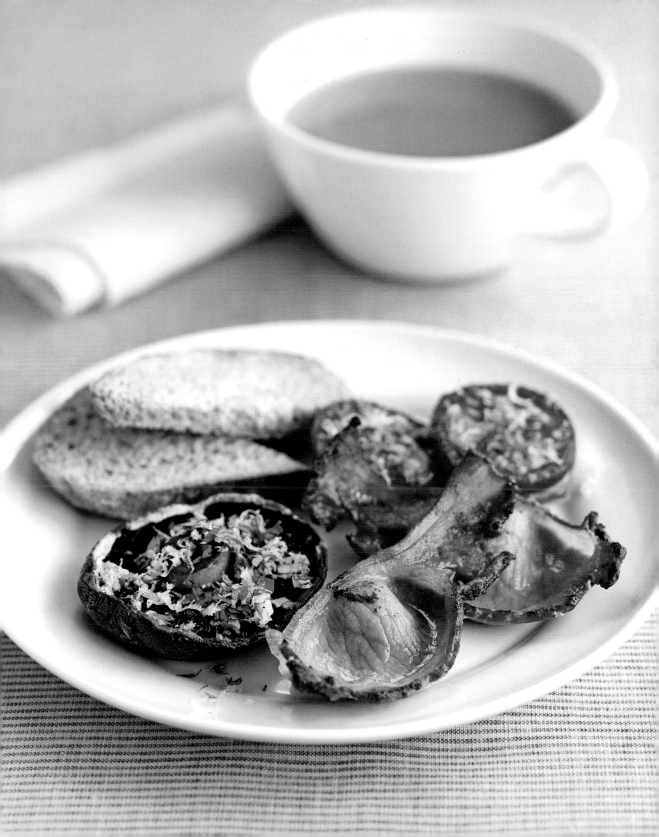

Poached egg and smoked trout on wholemeal toast

A truly scrumptious breakfast, this recipe is very quick, very tasty and very good for you. Always buy the best eggs you can afford. They really taste better, and you know those chickens are happier!

serves 1
prep time 5 minutes
cooking time 3–4 minutes
236 calories per serving

1 tablespoon vinegar
a pinch of salt
1 medium free-range egg
1 piece wholemeal toast
50g smoked trout
pepper

Fill a shallow pan (one that has a tight-fitting lid) with about 5cm water. Add the vinegar and a pinch of salt. Bring the water and vinegar mix to a boil, then turn it down to a tremble – just so the water is almost shivering. Crack your egg into a bowl.
Lower the egg into the simmering water and immediately put the lid on the pan and turn the heat off. Leave it like this for 3 minutes.
While the egg is poaching, make your toast. Arrange the layers of smoked trout on the toast and then top with your perfect poached egg. Add salt and pepper to taste.

Quick and easy kedgeree

Warming, exotic and yet oh, so comforting, this makes a great brunch or lunch dish (and as such, has a slightly higher calorie value than we recommend for breakfast). Hot-smoked salmon is widely available in supermarkets. Sold in vacuum-sealed packs, it has been cooked by the smoke rather than simply cured by it. Any leftover salmon can be flaked into salads or made into fishcakes.

serves 2
prep time 5 minutes
cooking time 15–20 minutes
346 calories per serving

vegetable oil spray
1 level teaspoon unsalted butter
¼ onion, finely chopped
100g basmati rice, rinsed
   and drained well
1 teaspoon mild, medium
   or hot curry powder
1 teaspoon ground turmeric

1 medium egg
75g hot-smoked salmon,
   flaked into chunks
1½ tablespoons flat-leaf parsley,
   chopped
a pinch of sea salt
a sprinkle of cayenne pepper
   (optional) to garnish

Try this with brown rice (bearing in mind that it will take longer to cook – check the packet instructions), and replace the parsley with chopped fresh coriander.

Heat the vegetable oil and butter and gently sauté the onion until just soft. Add the basmati rice and stir it for about 30 seconds, until it is coated with the oil and butter. Add the curry powder and turmeric and stir through the rice. Add 200ml cold water and bring to the boil. As soon as it is boiling, turn down to a very low heat and cover. Cook for about 10 to 12 minutes or until just cooked.

Put the egg into a pan of cold water to cover. Put the pan over the heat, and once the water is boiling, continue to cook for 3 to 4 minutes. Remove the egg from the pan and pop it into a cup of cool water. Check the rice is cooked and then take it off the heat. Let it sit with the lid on for 2 to 3 minutes to rest.

Gently stir the flaked salmon and half of the parsley into the rice. Put the lid back on for a minute or two, then taste and season with a pinch of salt if needed. (The salmon is salty, so you shouldn't need much.) Peel and quarter the egg carefully. Turn the kedgeree out onto plates and garnish it with the egg, the rest of the parsley and a sprinkle of cayenne pepper (optional).

Serve with a little yoghurt raita dressing (see page 217) on the side if you like.

Window-garden herb omelette

This is a really simple, quick and healthy option for breakfast or a lunch on the run. Whether you have a small flat or a big house, it's easy to manage a herb plant in a pot on the windowsill. Keep a couple of different ones, water them and snip off leaves to use as you require them. Our favourites – and ones that seem to thrive happily – are parsley, chives, chervil and basil.

serves 1
prep time 3 minutes
cooking time 4 minutes
171 calories per serving with Parmesan

2 free-range eggs
2 tablespoons fresh herbs from your windowsill, chopped
1 tablespoon Parmesan, freshly grated (optional)
vegetable oil spray
salt and pepper

Gently beat the eggs with a fork, just enough to combine them. Do not overbeat them. Add your choice of chopped herbs and, if using the Parmesan, add that too.
Spray 2 to 3 spritzes of oil into the pan and heat. Pour in the egg mixture and immediately start moving the outside layer of egg in by drawing it towards the middle with a spoon. As you do so, tilt the pan so that any runny egg finds its way into the gaps. Keep doing this until the egg is looking nicely cooked around the edges, but remains a little bit runny in the middle (not too runny – there shouldn't be any white that still looks clear or jelly-like).
Tilt your pan again, sliding the omelette onto your plate and folding it in half in one smooth movement. Season with salt and black pepper. Eat immediately.

Delicious served with roast cherry tomatoes on the vine, or with a green salad at lunchtime.

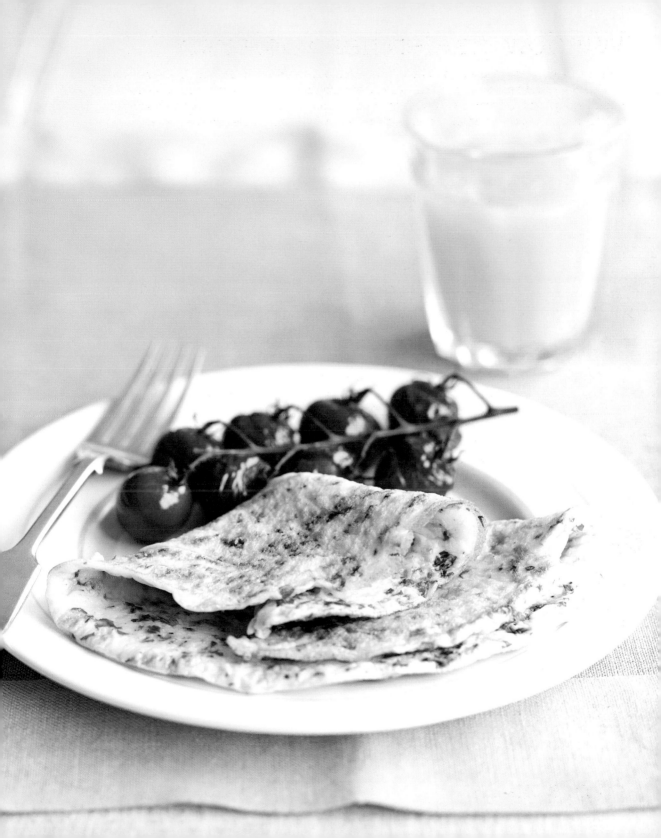

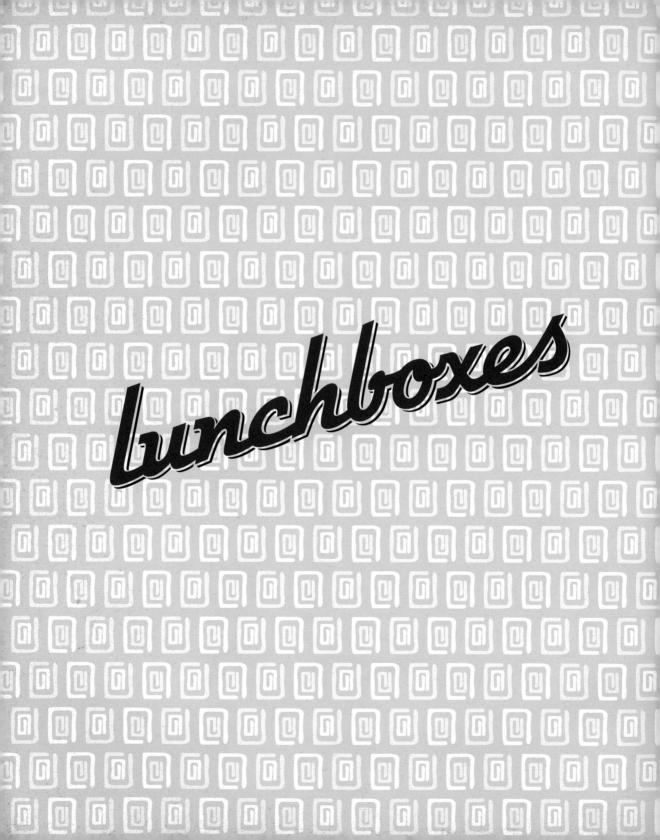

lunchboxes

We've packed our lunchboxes with skinny sandwiches, healthy wraps, slinky salads and a few little snacks to eat at home or take with you to work. Shop-bought sandwiches can be some of the worst offenders in the high-calorie stakes, so make your own lunch to give yourself an energy-packed, low-fat boost to the afternoon.

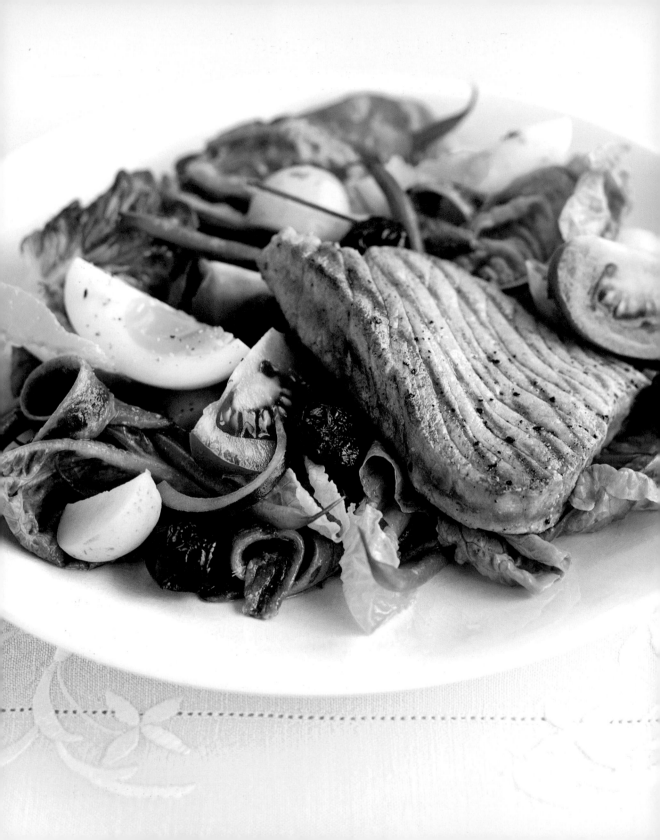

Seared fresh tuna Niçoise

This recipe takes the classic salade Niçoise and makes it super-healthy by cutting right back on the oil, using fresh tuna, and lightening the dressing.

serves 2
prep time 5 minutes
cooking time 10 minutes
310 calories per serving
322 calories per serving (with optional anchovies)

50g green beans, topped and tailed
1 tablespoon extra-virgin olive oil
1 tablespoon lemon juice
1 teaspoon Dijon mustard
1 teaspoon chopped fresh thyme leaves or ½ teaspoon dried thyme
mixed salad leaves of your choice
2 small tomatoes, quartered
1 small red onion, peeled and thinly sliced

6–8 small black olives, preferably wrinkly French Niçoise ones
4 tinned anchovies, drained and rinsed (optional)
200g tuna steak
extra-virgin olive oil spray
salt and freshly ground black pepper
1 egg
2 cooked new potatoes (leftover new potatoes are fine)

Blanch the green beans in boiling water for 2 minutes and refresh under cold water.

Mix the oil, lemon juice, mustard and thyme together to make a dressing. Set aside.

Place the leaves, tomatoes, onion, olives and the anchovies, if you're using them, in a big salad bowl. Mix everything together.

Heat a ridged griddle pan on the hob. Cut the tuna steak into two equal portions. Spritz it on both sides with 4 sprays of olive oil. Season with black pepper and a little salt, then grill on the hot griddle for 2 minutes on each side. Set the tuna aside to rest.

Put the egg in a pan of cold water, bring to the boil and cook for 5 to 6 minutes for a nice creamy yolk. Remove the egg immediately and put it in a bowl of cold water to stop it from cooking further.

Peel the egg and cut it into quarters along with the potatoes, then add the egg, potatoes and the green beans to the salad bowl. Pour over the dressing and toss the salad well.

Divide the salad between two bowls, place the tuna on top of the leaves and serve.

tip

Ring the changes by using chicken instead of tuna, replacing the lemon juice with a good wine vinegar, or using capers instead of the anchovies.

Sandwiches

For speed and convenience, you can't beat a sandwich. The problem is that so many of the sandwich shops pack their products full of mayonnaise and butter, and all too often, they only use a couple of kinds of bread. There are so many delicious different breads around now, making it easy to ring the changes and to pack more fibre and goodness into the humble sandwich: rye breads, black breads, wholemeal, sourdough and multi-grain all add loads of texture and flavour. Here are a couple of ideas to get you going. All these sandwich recipes serve one.

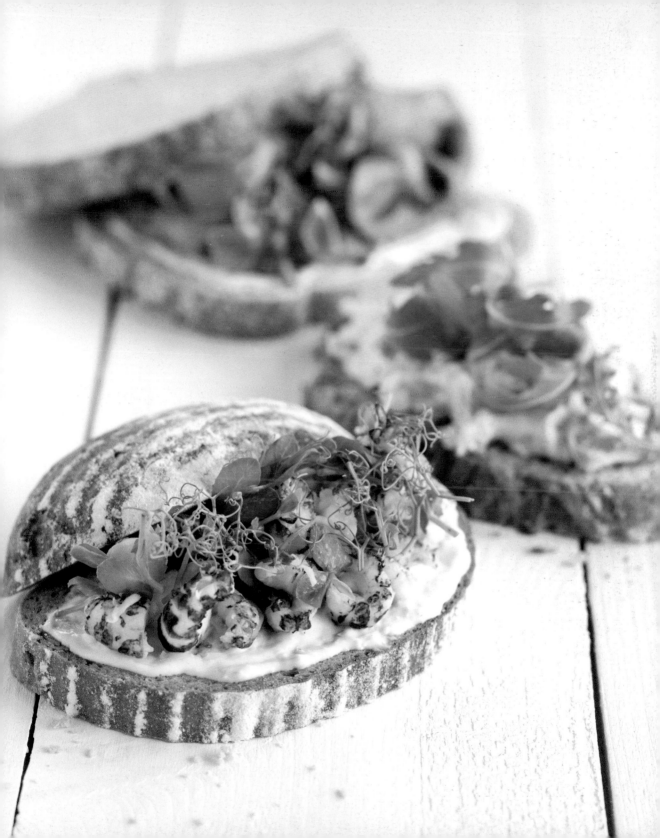

Rare beef with horseradish and watercress on wholemeal

A small confession here: if I'm served too much food at a restaurant, I always ask for a doggy bag to take it home in! So I'll occasionally find a beautifully cooked piece of rare steak lurking in my fridge, and thus this sandwich was born.

292 calories per serving
1 teaspoon ready-made horseradish sauce
1 teaspoon English mustard
1 teaspoon low-fat crème fraîche
2 slices of wholemeal bread
50g rare roast beef or steak, finely sliced
a handful of watercress

Mix the horseradish, mustard and crème fraîche together. Spread the mixture thinly onto wholemeal bread. Slice the beef as thinly as possible, and place on top of the horseradish mixture. Pile on the watercress and close the sandwich with another slice of wholemeal.

Lemony-garlic crayfish and pea shoots on rye

Pea shoots are fantastic! They have a delicious, sweet pea flavour with a nice soft salad crunch.

230 calories per serving
1 tablespoon low-fat crème fraîche
½ clove garlic, crushed
a good pinch of finely grated lemon zest
2 slices of rye bread
100g crayfish, thawed if frozen
a handful of pea shoots

Mix the crème fraîche, garlic and lemon zest together and smear thinly onto rye bread, then build your sandwich with the crayfish and pea shoots. Enjoy!

Peppery hot-smoked salmon open sandwich on granary bread

Hot-smoked salmon is delicious, and its flaky texture makes it work really well in this kind of sandwich.

372 calories per serving
50g hot-smoked salmon
1 tablespoon low-fat crème fraîche
freshly ground black pepper
a dash of green Tabasco
2 medium-cut slices of granary bread
a handful of wild rocket

Flake the salmon into the crème fraîche. Add the pepper and green Tabasco, and mix well. Smear onto the granary bread and cover generously with the rocket leaves.

Prawn and parsley couscous salad

We love couscous. It's so versatile, quick and delicious: couscous is a real store-cupboard must. If you leave out the prawns, this salad also goes beautifully with any grilled meats.

serves 4
prep time 10 minutes plus 15–20 minutes soaking
339 calories per serving

2 stoned dates or dried figs, chopped
juice of 1 orange
200g couscous
1 tablespoon extra-virgin olive oil
a large pinch of sea salt
¼–½ preserved lemon, depending on size, deseeded and chopped
a small bunch of flat-leaf parsley, chopped
1 tablespoon sultanas
300g cooked medium prawns
150g baby spinach, watercress and rocket salad (you can find this
    pre-mixed in bags in most supermarkets, or make your own blend)

Soak the dates or figs in the orange juice for 15 to 20 minutes.
While the fruit is soaking, pour 300ml boiling water over the couscous.
Add the extra-virgin olive oil and the sea salt and stir. Cover with a plate and leave to rest for 5 minutes.
Uncover the couscous and stir again. Add the drained fruit, sultanas, preserved lemon and parsley and stir well. Leave to cool for a few minutes and then stir through the prawns and the salad leaves.

You can easily make your own preserved lemons by slicing a couple of lemons in quarters almost through the fruit, but leaving it intact. Rub a tablespoon of sea salt into the cuts in each lemon and push them firmly into an empty jar with a tablespoon of sea salt, a dried chilli and a couple of cardamom pods in the bottom. Add the juice of 2 to 4 lemons to cover them. Shake the jar every day for a month. You now have lovely preserved lemons, which will keep for up to 6 months in the fridge, and a salty, spicy juice to use sparingly in salad dressings.

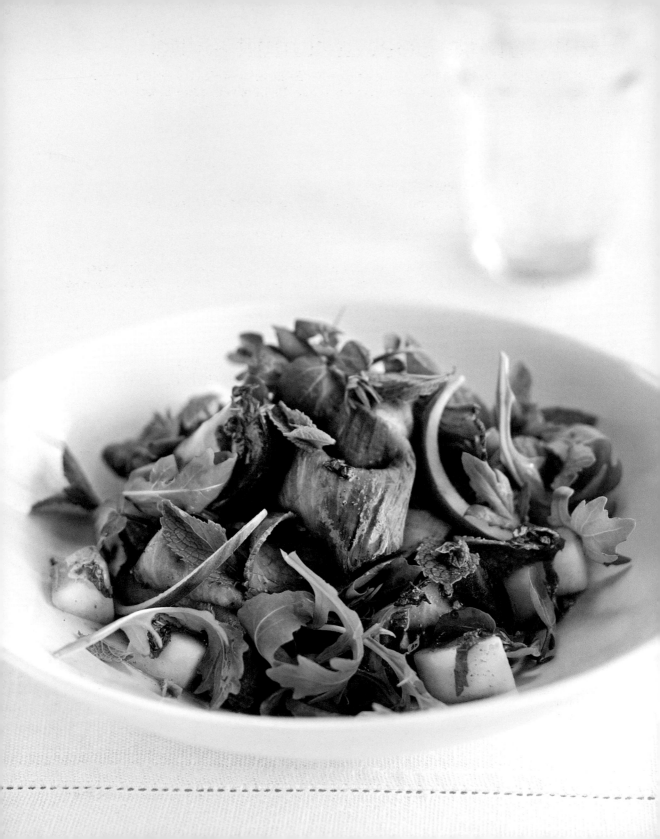

Vietnamese beef and mint salad

A quick, simple and delicious salad with a tangy Far-Eastern twist. This is a great way to use leftovers from the Sunday roast. You can substitute the beef with other meats – try pork, chicken, lamb or duck.

serves 2
prep time 10 minutes
cooking time 5–10 minutes (if cooking the beef from raw)
187 calories per serving
196 calories per serving (with optional ground rice)

200g beef (you could use leftovers or a nice piece of sirloin steak)
2 tablespoons nam pla (Thai fish sauce) or nuoc mam (its Vietnamese counterpart)
2 tablespoons lime juice
a pinch of sugar
¼ teaspoon pan-roasted chilli powder
1 teaspoon toasted ground rice (optional – see tip)
a bunch of mint leaves (about 20g), roughly chopped
½ cucumber, peeled and chopped
2 large or 4 small ripe tomatoes, quartered
½ red onion, thickly sliced
mixed salad leaves or the lettuce of your choice
lime, cut into wedges (optional)

If you're using leftover beef, just slice it into thin strips and set aside. If you're using fresh steak, lightly rub it with a teaspoon of extra-virgin olive oil and grill on a preheated ridged griddle pan over a medium flame. Cook for 2 minutes on each side for rare meat, or 3 to 4 minutes on each side for medium.
Take the steak off the griddle pan and let it rest whilst you whisk together the fish sauce, lime juice, sugar, chilli powder and toasted rice. Slice the steak into thin strips or gather your leftover beef, and pop it into the bowl with the dressing ingredients and half of the mint leaves.
Arrange the salad leaves on a plate with the cucumber chunks, tomatoes and onion.
Scatter the beef over the top, pour on the rest of the dressing and sprinkle over the rest of the mint leaves.
Serve with extra wedges of lime if you like!

tip

The toasted ground rice really makes a marked difference to the taste. You simply take a few tablespoons of raw, uncooked white rice and toast over a low to medium heat in a dry frying pan in a single layer for 4 to 5 minutes until golden brown and fragrant. Cool the rice and then either whiz in a food processor or use a pestle and mortar to grind it into a coarse powder. The rice powder can be kept in a screwtop jar or container for several months, ready to use whenever you make this salad.

Wraps

Wraps are so very easy: just warm up your chosen wrapper, spoon in a multitude of goodies and wrap everything up! Wraps are a great way to use up leftovers. You can make a multitude of delicious fillings by shredding any leftover salmon, chicken or meat, and mixing it with some of our dressing or dip ideas and lots of fresh salad. Delicious, healthy and economical – who could ask for more? All the wraps serve one unless otherwise stated.

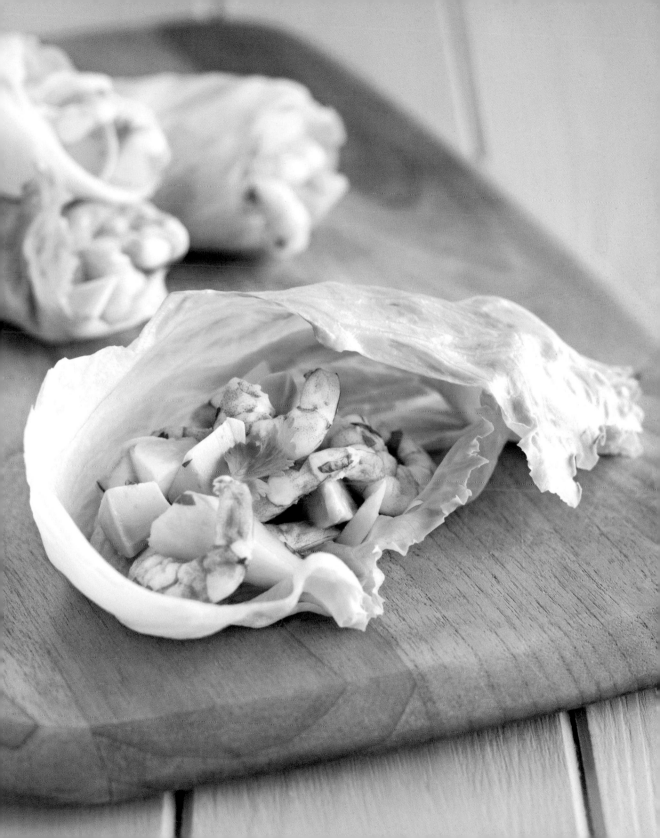

Prawn, avocado and mango wrap with coriander

A hint of the tropics. This no-bread wrap tastes so luxurious! Try crayfish tails, chunks of white crab meat or even lobster as a deluxe alternative. Papaya is also a great substitute for the mango. Using lettuce to wrap up the exotic filling instead of a flat bread wrapper makes this guilt-free!

serves 2
226 calories per portion
1 ripe mango, peeled, halved, stoned
    and cut into chunks
150g cooked, peeled prawns
1 small avocado, peeled, halved, stoned
    and cut into chunks
1 tablespoon chopped coriander
juice of ½ lime
a dash of Tabasco sauce
salt and pepper
½ iceberg lettuce or 2 baby gems

Mix the mango, prawns, avocado, coriander, lime juice and Tabasco in a large bowl, stirring well to combine all the ingredients. Season with a little salt and pepper. Divide the lettuce into leaves and place portions of the prawn mixture into each lettuce leaf, allowing 2 per person.

Club wrap

A sort of club sandwich – but healthier!

340 calories per portion
2 × 25g slices of turkey breast
1 Edam slice (pre-sliced packs are handy –
    each slice will weigh about 30g)
30g lettuce, shredded
1 small tomato, chopped
1 wrap of your choice
salt and freshly ground black pepper

Layer the turkey slices, cheese, lettuce and tomato in the wrap, season with salt and pepper and fold up. Yummy!

You can add a luxurious feel by spreading on 1 teaspoon of non-fat mayonnaise if you want, at the cost of only six calories. This wrap is great toasted in a sandwich press.

Wrap-around Manhattan

Brunch in New York City!

307 calories per portion
1 tablespoon non-fat cream cheese
50g smoked salmon
a squeeze of lemon juice
freshly ground black pepper
shredded iceberg lettuce
1 wholemeal wrap, warmed

Smear the non-fat cream cheese onto the wrap. Layer the smoked salmon over the top. Squeeze over the lemon and grind over some black pepper. Add the shredded lettuce, wrap up and enjoy!

Southern wild rice and Cajun chicken salad

Wild rice isn't actually rice at all, although it is closely related – it's a kind of grass seed. It is extremely nutritious, and has a lovely, nutty flavour.

serves 2
prep time 10 minutes
cooking time 45–50 minutes
344 calories per serving

2 × 100g skinless chicken breasts
extra-virgin olive oil spray
½ teaspoon cayenne pepper
½ teaspoon smoked paprika
¼ teaspoon sea salt
¼ teaspoon ground black pepper
a little grated nutmeg, to taste
1 dried bay leaf, stem removed
400ml water or chicken stock
50g wild rice
1 clove of garlic, peeled and
    crushed
1 teaspoon dried thyme

1 teaspoon dried oregano
salt and pepper
juice of ½ lemon
1 tablespoon extra-virgin olive oil
½ red or yellow pepper, deseeded
    and cut into chunks
2 sticks of celery, stringed and
    chopped
100g baby leaf spinach
4 spring onions, trimmed and
    chopped
2 tablespoons flat-leaf parsley,
    chopped

Make two diagonal slashes in the chicken breasts and spritz with oil. Pulverise the cayenne pepper, paprika, salt, black pepper, nutmeg and bay leaf, and pulverise using the back of a spoon or a pestle and mortar. Rub the chicken pieces all over with the mixture and leave to marinate. Bring the stock or water to a rolling boil and add the wild rice, garlic, thyme, oregano and a pinch of salt. Bring back to the boil and turn down to a simmer. Put the lid on and leave over a very low heat for about 50 minutes, until you can see the white interiors popping through the black skins of the grains, then drain and leave to cool.

Heat a ridged griddle pan over a low to medium heat and spritz with a few squirts of oil. Grill the chicken, for 7 minutes on each side. Check that it is cooked thoroughly – when the juices run clear, not pink, the chicken is ready. Remove it from the heat.

Mix the lemon juice, olive oil, salt and pepper together in a big bowl. Add the peppers, celery and baby spinach leaves, and toss. Add the rice, spring onion and parsley, and mix until coated. Adjust seasoning to taste. Slice the chicken into strips, place on top of the rice salad and serve.

tip

You can substitute fish or meat for the chicken. When buying chicken breasts, you will find it cheaper to buy them with the skin on. Just remove the skin yourself and throw it away.

Greek salad

The taste of this salad will take you right back to your holidays
– and it's so easy to make at home!

serves 2
prep time 10 minutes
217 calories per serving
359 calories served with 1 pitta bread per person

for the salad
80g feta cheese, cut into cubes
2 tomatoes, quartered
1 small red onion, sliced into thin rings
½ cucumber, peeled and cubed
8 black olives (preferably Kalamata), drained
for the dressing
1½ tablespoons extra-virgin olive oil
1 tablespoon lemon juice (more if you like it really sharp)
a pinch of salt
freshly ground black pepper
½ teaspoon dried oregano
½ tablespoon capers in brine or salt, rinsed (optional)

Take a large serving bowl and mix together the feta cheese,
tomato, red onion, cucumber and black olives.
Whisk the olive oil, lemon juice, salt and pepper, dried oregano
and the capers (if you're using them) together in a separate bowl.
Pour the dressing over the salad ingredients and mix well.

You can double
the dressing and
save half in a jar
in the fridge for use
later in the week.
A wholemeal pitta
bread is delicious
with this salad,
and will only add
142 calories.

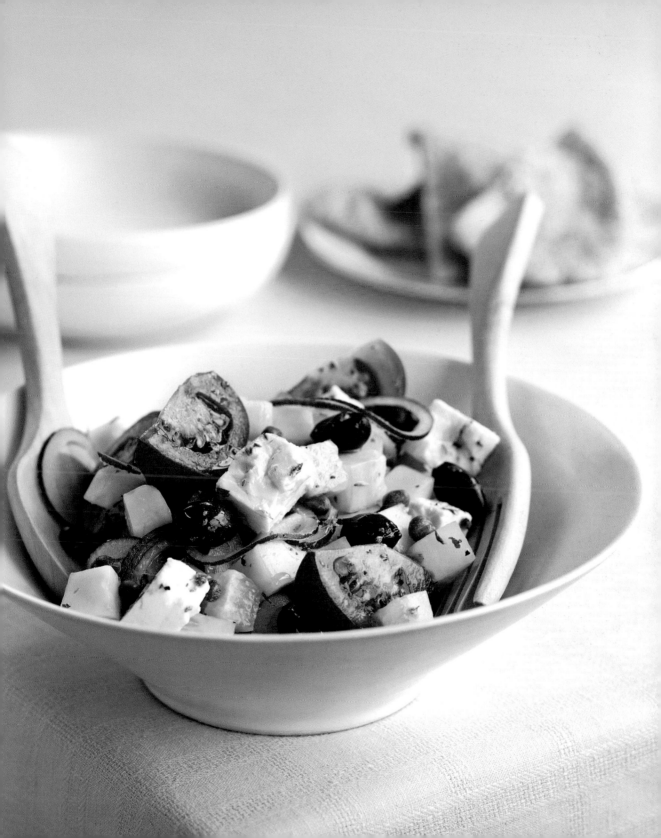

Zingy salad

This gives the lively flavour we love in a salad dressing, but without the lashings of olive oil found in traditional dressings. This recipe makes generous amount of dressing for two people, and will keep for a few days in the fridge.

serves 2
prep time 5 minutes
38 calories per serving

1 small unwaxed lemon
1½ teaspoons extra-virgin olive oil
1 tablespoon white balsamic vinegar
¼ teaspoon acacia blossom honey
green salad leaves

Grate the zest of the lemon into a jam jar.
Squeeze the lemon and add 2 tablespoons of the juice to the jar.
Add the olive oil, white balsamic vinegar and 1 teaspoon of water.
Finally, add the honey.
Put the lid on the jar and give it a good shake to emulsify the dressing.
Pour the dressing over the leaves and toss.

This is great with any green salad, but we also love it on a tuna and brown rice salad – healthy can be so tasty! See page 66 for the easy recipe.

Puy lentil and coriander salad

Healthy, and so very easy. Make a big batch of this and keep it in the fridge to go with grilled meats and fish.

serves 2
prep time 5 minutes
cooking time 20 minutes
304 calories per serving

150g Puy lentils
400ml vegetable stock or water
1 teaspoon ground coriander
salt and pepper
1 tablespoon lemon or lime juice
2 teaspoons extra-virgin olive oil
4 spring onions, trimmed and finely chopped
4 tablespoons coriander, chopped
2 fat beefsteak tomatoes, sliced
extra chopped coriander, for garnish

Rinse the lentils well, and pick through them to check for stones and dirt. Place them in a large saucepan with the vegetable stock.
Bring to the boil and then turn down to a simmer for 15 to 20 minutes until the lentils are cooked. Drain them. They should be al dente – like your pasta.
Mix together the ground coriander, salt, pepper, lemon juice and olive oil and pour over the lentils, mixing well.
Add the spring onions and the fresh coriander and stir gently. Serve over the sliced tomatoes.
Sprinkle with some more chopped coriander and serve.

For a change, try crumbling 100g feta cheese over the salad.

Tuna and brown rice salad

We've found this is a very popular dish to take to parties and barbecues – you'll always get to take home an empty bowl! It is a lovely summery dish, but the rice also makes it a substantial meal that will fill you up nicely.

serves 2
prep time 10 minutes
cooking time 25 minutes
255 calories per serving

100g brown short-grain rice
4 spring onions
1 pointy red pepper
80g albacore tuna in spring water from a jar or can, flaked
1 × zingy salad dressing (see page 64)

Cook the rice according to the packet instructions. Drain in a sieve and cool by running the sieve under the cold tap.
While the rice is cooking, chop the spring onions and the pepper and drain the tuna, reserving the spring water. Make up the zingy salad dressing, substituting the spring water from the tuna for the water in the recipe and adding a few drops of Tabasco sauce to taste.
Mix the cooled rice, spring onions, peppers, flaked tuna and salad dressing in a large bowl and serve.

You can use any kind of red pepper – we just really like the taste of the pointy ones!

To make this salad much more 'instant', you can cook up a big batch of rice and freeze it in portions, then just defrost what you need to make an instant scrummy meal, especially if you already have some salad dressing made up in the fridge (it can keep for up to a week).

Coronation chicken salad

This is a party for your taste buds! Super-quick and easy to make, this is one of those recipes that's destined to become a family favourite.

serves 2
prep time 5 minutes
cooking time 10 minutes
289 calories per serving

200g free-range chicken breast fillets, skinned and diced
extra-virgin olive oil spray
100g baby spinach
2 heaped tablespoons light mayonnaise
2 teaspoons medium curry powder
1 heaped teaspoon tomato puree
2 teaspoons fresh basil, roughly chopped
25g dried apricots, roughly chopped
25g sultanas
1 small crisp eating apple, cored and chopped into small cubes

Fry the chicken until nicely browned using a spritz of olive oil.
Divide the spinach between two plates to make a platform to lay the chicken on later.
In a large bowl, mix the mayonnaise, curry powder and tomato puree until they are combined.
Add all the other ingredients to the bowl and stir well until the fruit and chicken are coated.
Place a portion of the coronation chicken on top of the bed of spinach, and enjoy!

The recipe works fantastically if you add the chicken to the bowl whilst it is still warm, as long as you serve it immediately. It's also good with cold chicken, so we like to cook some diced chicken in batches and just keep it in the fridge for salads and recipes like this.

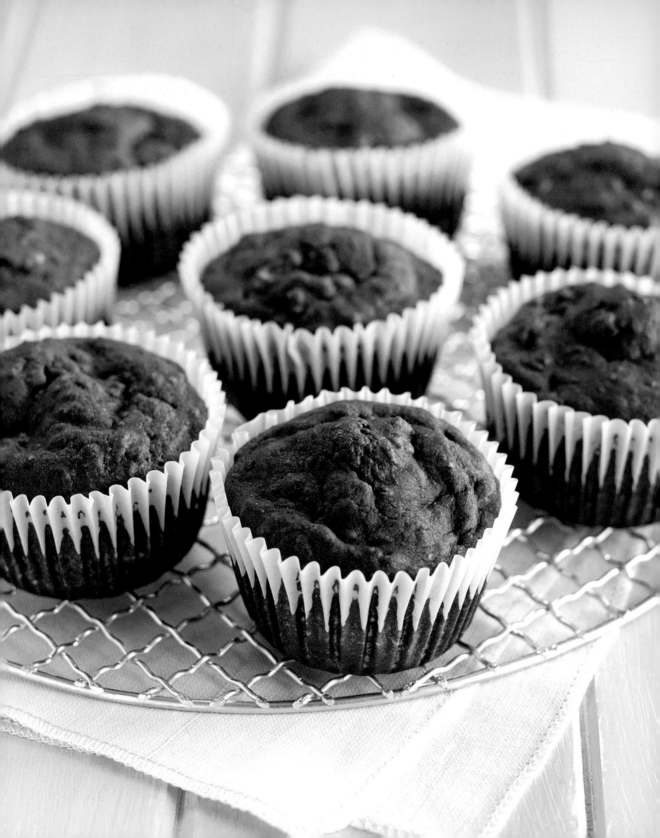

Chocolate-banana sunflower muffins

These are packed full of energy-boosting, feel-good ingredients that have excellent nutritional benefits. You will find it hard to believe that these guilt-free muffins are actually good for you!

makes 10–12 muffins
prep time 15 minutes
cooking time 15–18 minutes
154 calories per muffin (10 muffins)
145 calories per muffin (11 muffins)
133 calories per muffin (12 muffins)

50g spreadable light butter
50g dark chocolate (70% cocoa solids)
15g cocoa powder, sifted
25g rolled oats
25g spelt flour
1 medium egg
160g self-raising flour
40g caster sugar
25g pumpkin or sunflower seeds
1 teaspoon vanilla extract
½ teaspoon baking powder
50ml skimmed milk
1 ripe banana, mashed
150ml low-fat natural yoghurt

tip

If you like your muffins a little sweeter, try adding 2 tablespoons of honey to the milk mixture. (This will add calorie content – use your judgment. If you're preparing these for a lunchbox, where your calories should be kept low, you might prefer to leave the honey out.) Not a chocolate fan? They are just as lovely if you leave it out.

Preheat the oven to 200°C/fan 180°C.
Warm the butter and chocolate together in a pan over a gentle heat. Once melted, remove from the heat and allow to cool slightly.
Mix all the remaining ingredients together in a bowl, then add the chocolate mixture. Mix well, then spoon into a 10- to 12-hole muffin tray, or fill muffin cases. Bake for 15 to 18 minutes or until well risen and golden brown.
Cool on a wire tray, and then enjoy!

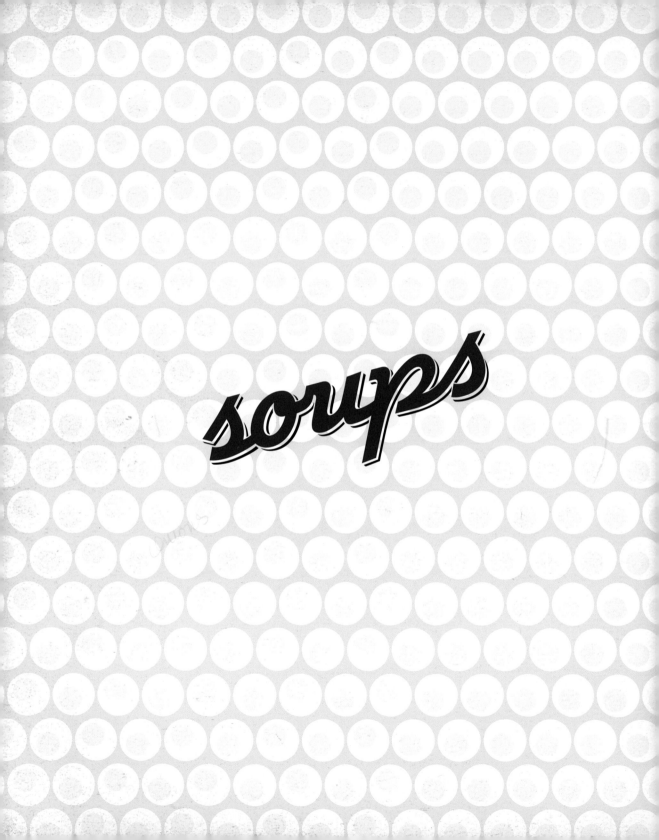

soups

Soups are one of the great secrets of Cooking Yourself Thin. Pick any one of the recipes here and you'll be giving yourself a really filling meal that's packed with goodness and low in calories. Make up a batch at the start of the week, freeze or refrigerate what's spare, and you'll have healthy, fast food whenever you need it – and no forks required!

French onion soup

This is a skinnier version of traditional French onion soup, with much less butter and alcohol, but hardly any difference in taste. The secret is in using home-made stock, or a pot of good ready-made stock from the supermarket. If you have beef stock, use it in preference to chicken stock – the soup will taste even better. Vegetarians can still enjoy this soup by simply replacing the stock and stock cube with vegetable varieties.

serves 3
prep time 10 minutes
cooking time 30 minutes
201 calories per serving

450g onions
1 tablespoon extra-virgin olive oil
1 clove of garlic
½ teaspoon granulated sugar
875ml beef, chicken stock or vegetable stock
    (preferably home-made)
1 beef or vegetable stock cube
75g baguette
1–2 teaspoons grated Parmesan cheese

Cut the onions in half and then into thin rings. (If your food processor has a slicing attachment, this can speed things up.)
Heat the olive oil in a large saucepan on the hob. Add the onion and garlic, and stir thoroughly to make sure they are coated in oil.
Add the sugar (this helps the onions caramelise) and stir. Keep stirring from time to time until the onions start to brown. This can take 10 minutes or longer; if you find the onions starting to catch on the bottom, just add a little stock and continue stirring, turning down the heat a little.
Keep stirring, and when the onions are golden-brown, add the stock. If you are vegetarian, just add water (this will bring the calorie count down by 30 calories per portion), or use a home-made vegetable stock. Add the stock cube. Bring to the boil and simmer for 20 to 30 minutes, or until the onions are really soft.
Toast one thick slice of baguette (2 to 3cm) per person. Sprinkle the toasted baguette with the Parmesan and melt under the grill.
Pour the soup into warm bowls and float the cheesy toast on top or serve alongside.

tip

One slice of cheesy baguette comes to 80 calories. If you want more, then add as many as your calorie allowance will permit. If you want to hand round extra Parmesan, then remember that each level tablespoon is only 40 calories.

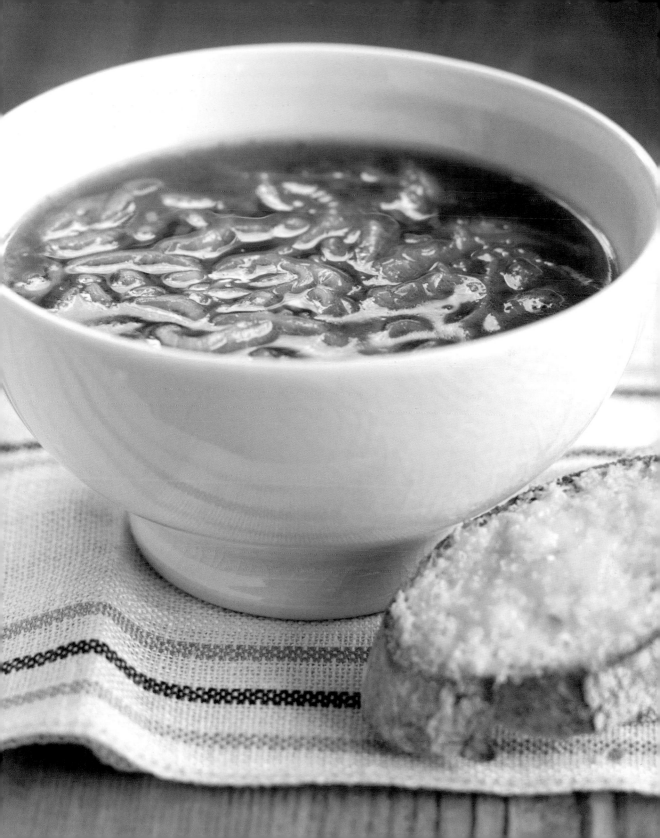

Hearty vegetable and lentil soup

This recipe is a great one to share with friends or eat on your own. It's low in fat, tasty and extremely filling. We love this soup because it's so versatile: you can add whichever vegetables you have available, using this recipe as a basis. Everyone who tries this asks for the recipe!

serves 4
prep time 10 minutes
cooking time 30 minutes
283 calories per serving

1 tablespoon extra-virgin olive oil
1 onion, finely sliced
3 cloves of crushed garlic
1½cm knob of ginger, peeled and minced
1 leek, sliced
2 large carrots, chopped
2 large potatoes, cut into 2½cm squares
100g red lentils
1 vegetable stock cube
5 dashes of Tabasco sauce (use more if you like it hotter!)
2 tablespoons Worcestershire sauce
1 tablespoon sherry vinegar
salt and freshly ground black pepper

Heat the olive oil in a large saucepan and gently fry the onion, garlic and ginger for 3 to 5 minutes, until the onion is just soft but not coloured.
Add the rest of the vegetables with the lentils and enough water to just cover the vegetables.
Simmer for 30 minutes or until the potatoes are cooked through.
Add the stock cube, Tabasco sauce, Worcestershire sauce and sherry vinegar. Stir thoroughly.
Season with salt and pepper to taste.
Serve in a soup bowl and tuck in.

tip

If a smooth texture is required, simply put the soup into a blender in batches, and whiz until they reach the required consistency. If you want it to be extra-smooth, you can use the back of a ladle to push the whizzed soup through a sieve.

Spicy Thai butternut squash soup

This soup is seriously low in calories, but tastes really indulgent. The amount of chilli can be adjusted to suit your personal taste.

serves 8
prep time 20 minutes
cooking time 30 minutes
119 calories per serving

extra-virgin olive oil spray
2 onions, chopped
2 chillies, deseeded and chopped
3 cloves of garlic, chopped
1½cm piece of ginger, peeled and finely chopped
2 lemongrass stalks, outer leaves removed, then chopped
1 large butternut squash (approx 1kg), peeled, deseeded and chopped
400ml can of reduced-fat coconut milk
1 vegetable stock cube
2 tablespoons nam pla (Thai fish sauce)
juice of 1 lime

Spritz a large saucepan eight times with olive oil. Add the onion, chilli, garlic, ginger and lemongrass to the pan and fry gently until the onion starts to soften.
Add the squash, coconut milk, stock cube, nam pla and enough boiling water to cover the squash.
Bring to the boil, covered, and simmer for approximately 20 minutes until the squash is soft.
Blend the soup until smooth with a hand blender or in a food processor. If you feel the soup is too thick, add some water. If you prefer a thicker texture, heat the blended soup and reduce it until it thickens.
Add the lime juice, stir well and serve piping hot.

tip

If you're in a hurry, you can buy pre-prepared ginger and lemongrass in jars.

Things on toast

Ah – toast, glorious toast! Perfect for those late-night moments after a long working day, when you need to eat something 'right this minute' and can't be bothered to cook. These toasts are super-quick, super-healthy and, most importantly, super-comforting.

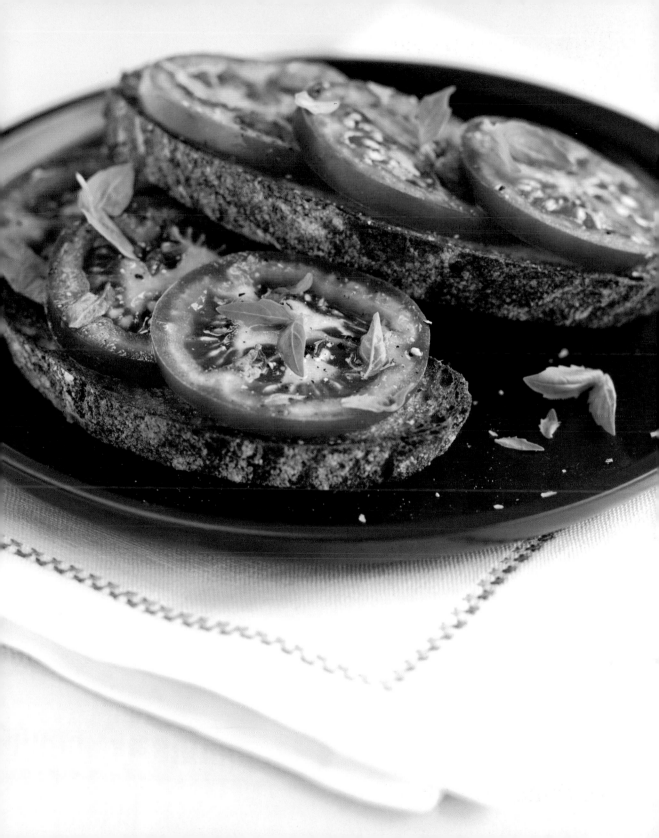

Tomato toast

Practically every European country has a recipe for this. From Spain to Malta, from to France to Turkey; the marriage of bread and tomatoes really works!

168 calories per serving
2 large or 4 small tomatoes, sliced
    or chopped
extra-virgin olive oil
a small handful of fresh basil, torn
sea salt and freshly ground black pepper
2 slices of sourdough bread
1 small clove of garlic, cut in half

Combine the tomatoes, a spritz of oil, the basil and salt and pepper to taste in a small bowl.
Toast the sourdough until golden.
Rub the cut side of the clove of garlic over the toast and top with the tomato mixture.

Marmite and avocado

Some people swear this tastes better with Bovril, but we are Marmite fans (you can try Vegemite as well). The avocado provides all the butteriness you need, as well as lots of vitamins and healthy fatty acids.

366 calories per serving
1 small avocado, peeled and sliced
    or chopped
a squeeze of lemon juice
2 slices of wholemeal bread
a little taste of Marmite – you know how
    much you like!
freshly ground black pepper

Slice or chop the avocado. Squeeze over a little lemon juice.
Toast the bread, and spread it with Marmite.
Layer the slices of avocado over the toast.
Season with freshly ground black pepper.

Sardines with cucumber, lemon and flat-leaf parsley

Always buy the best quality sardines (or Cornish pilchards) you can find – it makes a real difference.

249 calories per serving
½ × 120g tin of sardines in spring water
a dash of Worcestershire sauce, to taste
a squeeze of lemon juice
sea salt and freshly ground black pepper
1 spring onion, topped and tailed and finely
    chopped
2 teaspoons flat-leaf parsley, chopped
⅛ cucumber, peeled and finely chopped
2 slices of wholemeal or rye bread

Mash the sardines, removing the bones if necessary, with the Worcestershire sauce, a generous squeeze of lemon juice, sea salt and pepper.
Mix in the spring onion, parsley and cucumber. Stir to combine everything.
Make your toast and top with the sardine mixture. Eat while the toast is hot and crisp.

Sweet potato and apple soup

This is a deliciously warming, filling soup that tastes luxurious but has few calories.
It's great for lunch – try taking some to work in a Thermos.

serves 4
prep time 10 minutes
cooking time 25 minutes
143 calories per serving

1 tablespoon extra-virgin olive oil
1 onion, finely chopped
420g peeled sweet potatoes, diced into 1½cm pieces
1cm piece of ginger, peeled
1 teaspoon cumin seeds
1 teaspoon ground coriander
140g Bramley apples, peeled, cored and diced into 1.5cm pieces
salt and freshly ground black pepper

Heat the oil in a pan, and gently fry the onion for 5 minutes until
soft, but not browned.
Add the sweet potato, ginger, cumin, coriander and apple. Cover
with about 750ml boiling water.
Bring to the boil, then turn down the heat and simmer with the lid
on for 20 minutes until the sweet potato is tender.
Whiz with a hand blender or in the food processor until the soup
is smooth. Season to taste and serve.

This soup tastes
fantastic garnished
with a scattering
of fresh coriander.

Maltese pea and cumin soup

Ah! The taste of a sunny Mediterranean day. This is based on the flavours of the traditional Maltese pea cake or *pastizzi*, but uses fresh (frozen) peas instead of dried split peas.

serves 2
prep time 5 minutes
cooking time 10 minutes
156 calories per serving

2 teaspoons cumin seeds
extra-virgin olive oil spray
1 clove of garlic, peeled and sliced
2 teaspoons ground cumin
500ml vegetable or chicken stock
400g frozen peas
salt and pepper

Heat a dry, non-stick pan over a low heat and toast the cumin seeds for a few minutes until fragrant and golden. Remove from the heat and set aside.
Spritz a heavy-based saucepan with some of the olive oil spray. Heat gently over a very low heat and sauté the garlic gently until soft but not brown.
Add the ground cumin and stir for another minute.
Pour the stock into the pan and bring to the boil. Add the frozen peas, bring back to the boil and simmer for 5 minutes. Season with salt and pepper.
Ladle the soup into a blender (careful – it'll be hot!) and whiz until smooth, or puree with a hand blender. Taste, and adjust the seasoning. Serve hot or cold, scattered with the toasted cumin seeds.

tip

Frozen peas are a lifesaver – and so healthy! It's a good idea to keep a bag or two in the freezer. Make soups, rough purées for dipping crudités into, or mix with low-fat yoghurt and mint to make a fresh, light dressing for a Jersey Royal potato salad. Some of the supermarkets now stock pea shoots in their salad sections, and they're delicious scattered on top of this soup as well.

Speedy gazpacho

So light and refreshing in the summer! If you want to glam this up to serve to friends, pour into pretty tea glasses or vintage cups and add a dash of vodka too!

serves 1
prep time 10 minutes
cooking time 5 minutes
183 calories per serving

2 large, juicy tomatoes, peeled
1 clove of garlic, peeled and chopped
1 small slice of white bread (19g), torn into pieces
1 teaspoon extra-virgin olive oil
1 teaspoon red wine vinegar
125ml iced water
salt and pepper
a few dashes of Tabasco sauce
a dash of Manzanilla or other dry sherry (optional)
¼ red pepper, deseeded and diced
¼ green pepper, deseeded and diced
1 small mild red onion, finely diced

Pop the tomato, garlic, bread, olive oil and the wine vinegar into a blender and whiz.
Add the iced water and stir well.
Pour the gazpacho into a bowl or pretty glass, and add salt, pepper, Tabasco to taste and the sherry too, if you're using it. Add the diced red and green peppers and the diced red onion.

Roast beetroot and apple soup

A healthy and delicious take on traditional borscht. For an extra treat, you could cut 25g feta cheese into cubes, and sprinkle them on top of the soup.

serves 2
prep time under 10 minutes
cooking time 40 minutes
114 calories per serving

300g raw beetroots, peeled and quartered
1 small onion, finely chopped
a large sprig of thyme
1 large eating apple, peeled, cored and quartered
vegetable oil spray
500ml vegetable or chicken stock
salt and freshly ground black pepper
1 tablespoon flat-leaf parsley, chopped

Preheat the oven to 200°C/fan 180°C.
Place the beetroot, onion, thyme and apple in a roasting tin. Spritz them lightly with oil and season with salt and pepper. Cover with a sheet of foil. Roast for 30 to 40 minutes, testing with a knife after 30 minutes. The fruit and beets should be soft, giving easily to the knife. Remove them from the oven and set aside.
Heat the stock over a gentle flame until it comes to a simmer. Add the beetroot, apple and thyme, and bring back to the boil. Add salt and freshly ground black pepper.
Take the soup off the heat, remove the sprig of thyme and pour carefully into a blender or use a hand blender. Whiz the soup until it is smooth. Taste and adjust the seasoning.
Serve hot or cold with a sprinkle of parsley. Season to taste.

tip
If you manage to find beetroots with the leaves still on, don't throw them away. The leafy parts are very delicious served as a green vegetable or even made into a soup themselves. You could add 1 tablespoon of half-fat crème fraîche (65 calories) to the soup just before serving.

82 soups

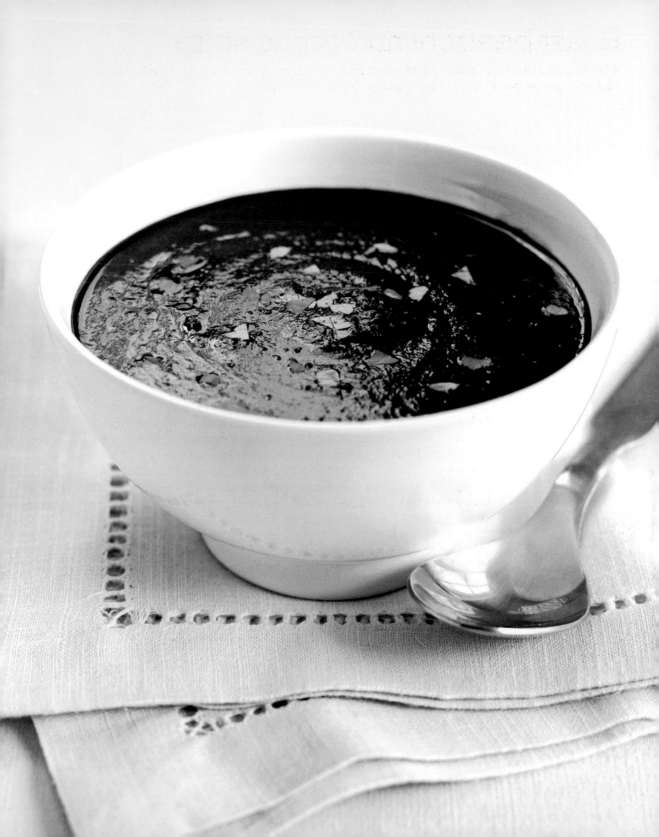

Spiced carrot and orange soup

Bright and sunny as a summer's day – with tons of vitamins too!

serves 2
prep time 10 minutes
cooking time 20 minutes
113 calories per serving

extra-virgin olive oil spray
½ onion, chopped
1 clove of garlic, peeled and chopped
½ teaspoon ground cumin
1 teaspoon ground coriander
½ teaspoon mild or hot curry powder
juice of 1 large orange
600ml vegetable stock
400g carrots, peeled and chopped
salt and pepper

Spritz a heavy-based saucepan a couple of times with olive oil.
Heat the pan and gently sauté the onion and garlic until soft. Add the
ground cumin, ground coriander and curry powder, and stir until
fragrant. Add half of the orange juice and allow to bubble for 1 minute.
Add the stock and bring to the boil. Add the carrots and simmer, covered,
until they are soft and cooked through, about 20 minutes. Check and give
them more time if they need it. Add salt and pepper to taste. Add the
other half of the orange juice. Taste, and adjust the seasoning.
Pour carefully into a food processor or use a hand blender, and whiz
until the soup is nice and smooth.
Serve hot with a dusting of ground cumin and coriander.

If you have some
friends coming
round, serve this
soup in tiny egg or
sake cups for a filling
yet healthy *amuse
bouche*. Very posh!

Jerusalem artichoke soup

We love the fact that these gnarled, knobbly looking vegetables produce a soup that tastes so rich and creamy, without having a single drop of dairy in it. Jerusalem artichokes grow prolifically in Britain. If you cannot find them in your supermarket, find a nearby allotment – they will be giving them away!

serves 2
prep time 15 minutes
cooking time 30–40 minutes
119 calories per serving

extra-virgin olive oil spray
2 cloves of garlic, peeled and sliced
500ml chicken or vegetable stock
2 sprigs of thyme
450g Jerusalem artichokes, scrubbed and peeled
    and cut into chunks
salt and pepper

Soften the garlic over a very low heat in a heavy-based saucepan spritzed with olive oil.
Add the stock and the thyme and bring to the boil. Add the Jerusalem artichokes, bring back to the boil and simmer for about 30 minutes until they are soft.
Pour carefully into a blender or use a hand blender to whiz the soup until it is smooth. Season to taste with salt and pepper, and serve piping hot.

Try substituting celeriac for Jerusalem artichokes. For another twist, you could roast the Jerusalem artichokes or celeriac or do a combination of both.

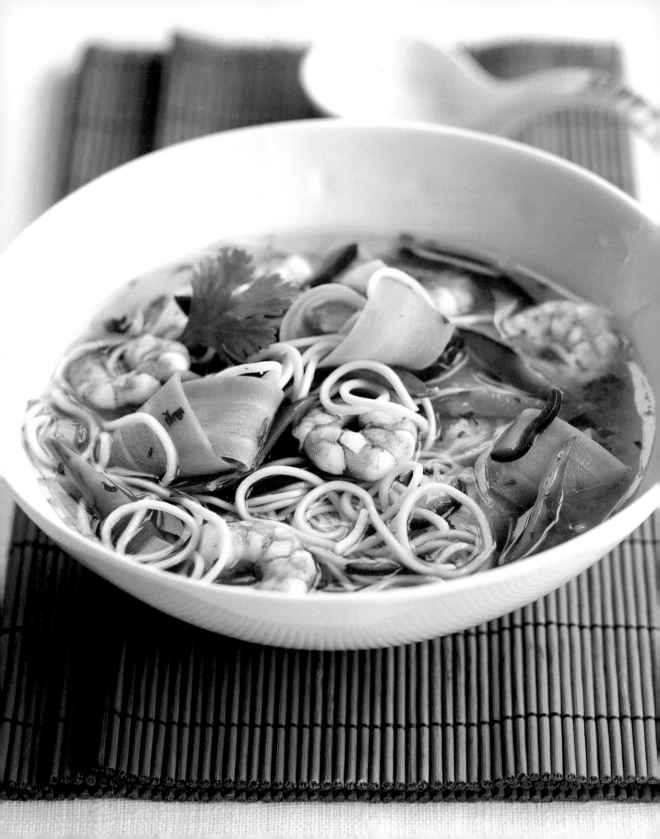

Hot-and-sour prawn noodle soup

Sweet, tart and spicy, this soup comes in a huge portion that is bound to fill you up.

serves 2–3
prep time 15 minutes
cooking time 30 minutes
385 calories per serving (if serving 2)
257 calories per serving (if serving 3)

1 teaspoon sunflower oil
1 medium onion, chopped
2 cloves of garlic, chopped
1cm piece of ginger, peeled
   and finely sliced
2 medium carrots, peeled
2 red chillies, thinly sliced
½ teaspoon salt
1 tablespoon dark soy sauce
100g fine egg noodles

juice of 1 lime
1 tablespoon nam pla
   (Thai fish sauce)
½ medium red pepper,
   thinly sliced
100g mange tout, raw
200g raw king prawns, peeled
25g coriander leaves, finely
   chopped

Heat the oil in a large, non-stick saucepan, and gently fry the onion, garlic, ginger, one of the carrots (chopped), and half the chilli for around 3 to 4 minutes.

Add 800ml water from the kettle to the pan with the salt and soy sauce, and bring everything to a rolling boil. Reduce the heat and simmer for 10 minutes.

While the stock is simmering, boil the noodles in a pan of salted water for 2 minutes, drain and set aside. Use a vegetable peeler to cut the remaining carrot into ribbons.

Once the stock is cooked, sieve it into a large wok, making sure you push all the juices out of the vegetables before discarding them. Bring the stock to a simmer again and add the lime juice, fish sauce and the rest of the chilli with the red pepper, mange tout and carrot ribbons. Simmer gently for 3 minutes.

After 3 minutes, add the cooked noodles and prawns. Stir well and continue to simmer for 2 to 3 minutes.

Once the prawns are pink and firm, add the coriander and serve immediately in large bowls with a spoon and chopsticks.

tip

This soup is very spicy, so if you want you can remove the chilli seeds or simply use a smaller amount of chilli.

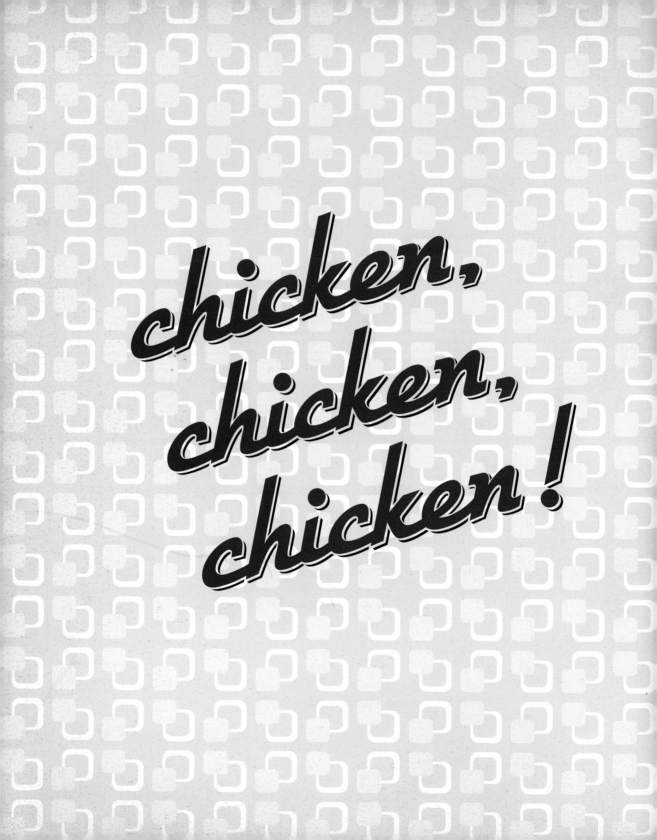

It seems we're all mad about chicken. Some of us are eating it as much as three or four times a week, but we tend to cook the same old dishes and we're sick of them! Chicken is a great source of protein and is generally low in fat once the skin has been removed. The recipes here are a mixture of tasty twists on old favourites and new ideas to try out.

Catalan chicken

A rustic, hearty Mediterranean dish, perfect for sharing with friends or family.

makes 4 servings
prep time 15 minutes
cooking time 45 minutes
302 calories per serving

1 tablespoon extra-virgin olive oil
3 large cloves of garlic, roughly chopped
1 Spanish onion, chopped
2 sticks of celery, roughly chopped
1 Romano pepper, deseeded and cut into strips
50g serrano ham, sliced into ribbons
extra-virgin olive oil spray
4 × 100g chicken thighs
125ml Manzanilla sherry
1 tablespoon sherry vinegar
500ml chicken stock (preferably home-made)

a handful of rosemary, thyme and flat-leaf parsley, chopped
a good pinch of saffron, soaked in an egg cup of hot water
1 small (230g) tin of chopped tomatoes
2 teaspoons ground paprika
2 thick strips of orange zest
salt and pepper
1 tin (410g) of borlotti, cannellini or butter beans, drained and rinsed
1 tablespoon finely chopped flat-leaf parsley
2 teaspoons finely grated orange zest

Heat the olive oil in a heavy-based wide pan over a very low heat. Sauté the garlic, onion, celery and pepper for a few minutes until softened. Remove the vegetables and set aside. Add the serrano ham and carry on sautéing for a few minutes. Remove from the pan and set aside. Add a spray of olive oil to the pan and brown the chicken. Set aside. Place the pan back on the heat and pour in the sherry and the sherry vinegar, scraping at the sides to deglaze all the yummy bits stuck to the bottom, and bring to the boil. Add the stock and bring to the boil. Put the chicken, vegetables and ham back in the pan and bring back to a simmer. Add the handful of fresh herbs, the saffron and its water, the tomatoes, paprika, orange zest strips, salt and pepper. Bring back to the boil, reduce the heat, and cover and simmer for 10 minutes. Now remove the lid and let the chicken simmer gently for another 20 minutes. Add the beans and simmer for another 5 minutes. Taste and adjust the seasoning.
Garnish with the parsley and grated orange zest.

tip

We love to make our own chicken stock. It tastes better, you can control exactly what goes into it, and it's economical too!

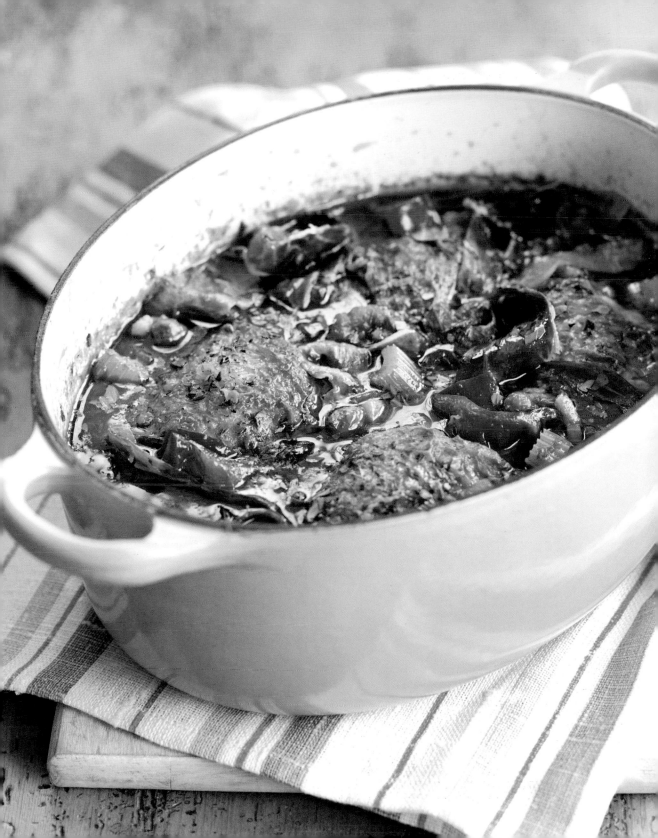

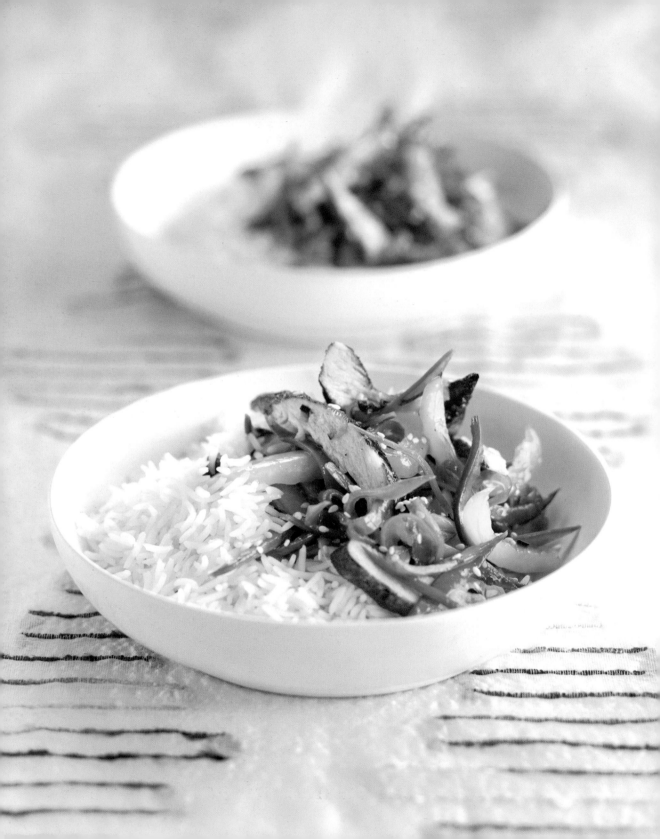

Five-spice chicken with a vegetable stir-fry

This low-cal chicken dish is really simple to create, but looks like you have spent hours in the kitchen – perfect for when you are entertaining friends, but would rather enjoy their company than that of your pots and pans. Lovely!

serves 4
prep time 10 minutes
cooking time 25 minutes
219 calories per serving
399 calories per serving with 50g raw rice per portion

1 heaped tablespoon
   sesame seeds
2 teaspoons five-spice powder
400g free-range chicken
2 teaspoons toasted sesame oil
1 tablespoon vegetable oil
6 spring onions, sliced
1 clove of garlic, crushed
1 red chilli, deseeded and
   finely chopped

110g mange tout, shredded
90g baby leaf spinach, chopped
1 yellow pepper, deseeded
   and sliced
1 tablespoon clear honey
2 tablespoons dark soy sauce
2 tablespoons plum sauce
2 tablespoons fresh coriander,
   chopped

tip

To cook perfect rice for four, put 200g basmati rice and a pinch of salt in a saucepan. Pour over enough water to cover the rice by 1cm. Bring to the boil and simmer for 8 minutes, covered. Remove from the heat and leave, covered, to absorb the remaining water for 10 minutes.

Preheat the oven to 200°C/fan 180°C.
Toast the sesame seeds in a dry frying pan until pale golden brown.
Sprinkle the five-spice onto a plate and rub the chicken pieces in it until they are well coated.
Heat a griddle pan and grill the chicken until it is seared.
Remove the chicken from the pan, place on a baking tray and cook in the oven for 15 minutes until cooked through.
Meanwhile, heat the oil in a wok or large frying pan, add the spring onion, garlic and chilli and stir fry for 2 minutes. Add the mange tout and spinach and cook for a further 1 to 2 minutes. Add the pepper, then stir in the honey.
Add the soy sauce and plum sauce and cook for a further 2 minutes until the sauce thickens slightly.
Stir in the chopped coriander and sesame oil. Remove from the heat.
Slice the chicken, mix with the stir-fried vegetables and serve over a bed of boiled rice sprinkled with the toasted sesame seeds.

Creamy chicken curry

Leftover chicken from a Sunday roast and stock made from the chicken carcass make a quick and creamy curry packed with flavour. Butternut squash is a Cook Yourself Thin favourite, and makes this curry even richer – and amazingly low in calories!

serves 4
prep time 15 minutes
cooking time 35 minutes
185 calories per serving
365 calories per serving with 50g raw rice per portion

½ teaspoon extra-virgin olive oil
2 onions, chopped
1 clove of garlic, crushed
1 teaspoon sea salt
200g butternut squash, peeled, deseeded and cut into 1cm cubes
4 stalks of celery, sliced
1 red pepper, deseeded and chopped
280g leftover roast chicken, cut into bite-sized pieces
1 heaped teaspoon medium curry powder
½ teaspoon ground ginger
1 teaspoon ground turmeric
300ml chicken stock (make your own from the roast chicken carcass)
50g half-fat crème fraîche
a handful of chopped coriander

If you don't have much leftover chicken, try adding extra vegetables instead. Just use whatever you have in your garden, cupboard or fridge. A home-made stock tastes best in this recipe, but if you haven't had time to make some, buy fresh stock at the supermarket.

Take a non-stick frying pan and wipe the olive oil around the surface. Add the onion, garlic, sea salt and butternut squash, and fry gently to soften, stirring occasionally, for about 5 minutes.
Add the celery and pepper to the pan and fry for another couple of minutes. Add the chicken pieces and curry powder, the ginger and the turmeric. Stir gently for a minute to make sure the flavours mingle, then gradually add the chicken stock, stirring all the time.
Simmer for 40 minutes or until the squash is very tender, but retains its cube shape. Stir in the crème fraîche.
Sprinkle the coriander leaves over the curry and serve with boiled rice – see the tip on page 93 for a quick and easy rice method.

Tarragon chicken

This recipe takes no time at all to prepare, and tastes much richer than it actually is. Tarragon chicken is a great supper dish for those evenings when you're short on time. Try serving with a crispy salad and crusty bread, or some rice to mop up the creamy sauce.

serves 2
prep time 10 minutes
cooking time 15 minutes
326 calories per serving

2 × 100g skinless free-range chicken breasts
salt and pepper
1 tablespoon extra-virgin olive oil
100ml chicken stock
200ml half-fat crème fraîche
2 tablespoons chopped fresh tarragon (or 1 tablespoon dried)
1 tablespoon chopped fresh coriander
½ tablespoon Dijon mustard
1 tablespoon lemon juice

Chop the chicken breasts into bite-sized pieces, and season with salt and pepper.

Heat the oil in a sauté pan. Place the chicken pieces into the pan and sauté until cooked through, turning constantly so that the chicken doesn't burn but is nicely golden-brown on all sides. Don't overcook the chicken, or it will be dry. Turn down the heat to low.

Add the chicken stock. When it starts to bubble, tip in the crème fraîche, herbs, mustard and lemon juice and bring to a low simmer. Taste to see if it needs any more seasoning.

Serve immediately with a crispy salad and crusty bread or, if you want something a little more substantial, with rice and a side salad.

tip

Vegetarians can try using Quorn pieces instead of chicken, for even fewer calories!

Creamy lemon-coriander chicken curry with red peppers

A great curry to cook for friends or just as a treat for yourself, this is simple to prepare and tastes deliciously creamy and zingy without actually contributing to your waistline. The cream is replaced with natural yoghurt, and the spices and garlic provide antioxidants.

serves 6
prep time 20 minutes
cooking time 1 hour 20 minutes
228 calories per serving
408 calories per serving with 50g raw rice per portion

3 cloves of garlic, finely chopped
2 large onions, finely chopped
1 tablespoon olive oil
1 teaspoon cumin seeds
3 cardamom pods
1 teaspoon ground turmeric
1 teaspoon chilli powder, mild to hot
1 red pepper, deseeded and roughly chopped
1 teaspoon concentrated chicken bouillon or vegetable stock powder
25g fresh coriander, roughly chopped
650g cooked free-range chicken, diced, without skin
150g low-fat natural plain yoghurt
juice and grated zest of ½ lemon
salt and pepper

tip

Once the chicken has been added, the curry can be cooked slowly for up to 2 hours, depending on when you wish to serve it. Plan the rice around the end of the curry's cooking time, and be sure to add the yoghurt right at the last moment. See the tip on page 93 to learn how to cook perfect rice.

Fry the garlic and onion in the olive oil in a large saucepan until translucent. Add the cumin, cardamom pods, turmeric and chilli powder, adding water instead of oil if anything starts to stick. Cook for 2 minutes. Add the red pepper, bouillon or stock powder and enough water to cover the ingredients. Add half of the coriander and simmer over a low heat until the red pepper is soft.

Stir the chicken into the pan until heated through. Add the lemon juice, stir, and leave over a low heat for at least half an hour, until the chicken has become tender and the peppers have begun to break down. Take off the heat and stir in the yoghurt, reserving 1 tablespoon for serving. Once the chicken is tender, stir in most of the remaining coriander and all the lemon zest, reserving a little coriander to garnish. For an optional extra indulgence, add a splash of cream. Season to taste.

Serve piping hot with boiled rice and season with the remaining dollop of yoghurt and coriander.

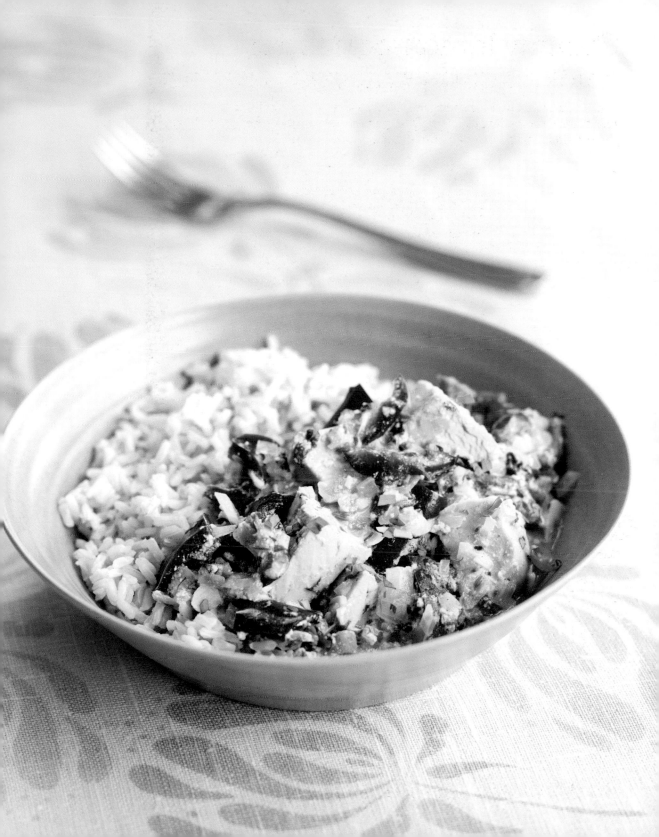

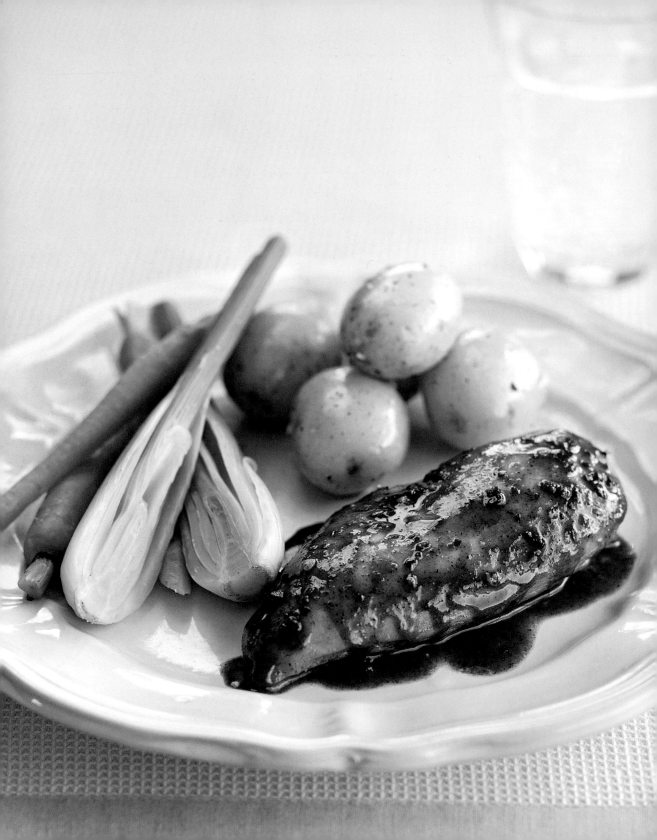

Maple syrup chicken

This dish is great either on the barbecue in summer or in the oven in winter.
It has a lovely sweet flavour, so it feels really naughty!

serves 2
prep time 5 minutes plus 2 hours marinating
cooking time 35 minutes
196 calories per serving
376 calories per serving with 50g raw rice per portion

2 tablespoons maple syrup
1 tablespoon soy sauce
juice of 1 lemon
1 clove of garlic, crushed
½ teaspoon dried chilli flakes
½ teaspoon ground paprika
½ teaspoon ground nutmeg
2 × 100g skinless free-range chicken breasts
salt and freshly ground black pepper

Mix all the ingredients together and marinate the chicken in a sealed,
non-metallic container for a minimum of 2 hours and preferably all day
or overnight.
Preheat the oven to 180°C/fan 160°C.
Place the chicken, reserving the marinade, in a deep baking tray.
Cover loosely with foil and bake for 30 to 35 minutes.
In a small saucepan, bring the reserved marinade to the boil and
simmer for approximately 5 minutes. The sauce should reduce right
down to between a half and a third of the original amount.
Serve by pouring the sauce over the top of the chicken. This goes well
with boiled rice (page 93), or four to six egg-sized new potatoes and
baby vegetables.

Harissa-spiced chicken with bean and couscous salad

A simple and quick chicken recipe that takes very little effort, but delivers maximum flavour.

serves 2
prep time 15 minutes
cooking time 10 minutes
396 calories per serving

for the chicken
2 × 100g skinless free-range
  chicken breasts
1 tablespoon harissa
  (we like Belazu rose harissa)
1 tablespoon runny honey
juice of ½ lemon
½ teaspoon ground coriander
½ teaspoon ground cumin
½ teaspoon ground cinnamon
1 teaspoon extra-virgin olive oil

for the couscous
100g couscous
1 spring onion, finely chopped
125ml chicken stock
juice of ½ lemon
½ can of mixed beans, drained
1 tomato, seeded and diced
1 tablespoon fresh mint, chopped
salt and freshly ground black pepper
to serve
1 tablespoon low-fat natural yoghurt

Slice the chicken breasts in two lengthways to give you four thinner pieces (this will allow them to cook quickly). Slash each fillet twice to a depth of 1cm.

Mix the harissa, honey, lemon juice, spices and oil together in a non-metallic bowl, and allow the chicken to marinate in this mixture for as long as you have (try to leave it in the mixture for at least 20 minutes. If you have time, marinate it overnight).

Put the couscous in a bowl with the chopped spring onion and pour over the hot chicken stock and lemon juice. Cover and leave to stand for 5 minutes.

Fluff up the couscous with a fork, then add the beans, diced tomato and chopped mint. Season to taste, mix well and cover again until ready to use.

Heat a non-stick frying pan or griddle over a medium heat. Add the chicken breasts and cook until lovely and caramelized on the outside and cooked through in the middle; about 4 minutes on each side.

Serve two pieces of chicken on top of a generous pile of couscous. Finish with a drizzle of natural yoghurt.

tip

Don't panic if the chicken starts to blacken a little; it's just the honey in the marinade caramelising, which adds flavour.

100 chicken, chicken, chicken!

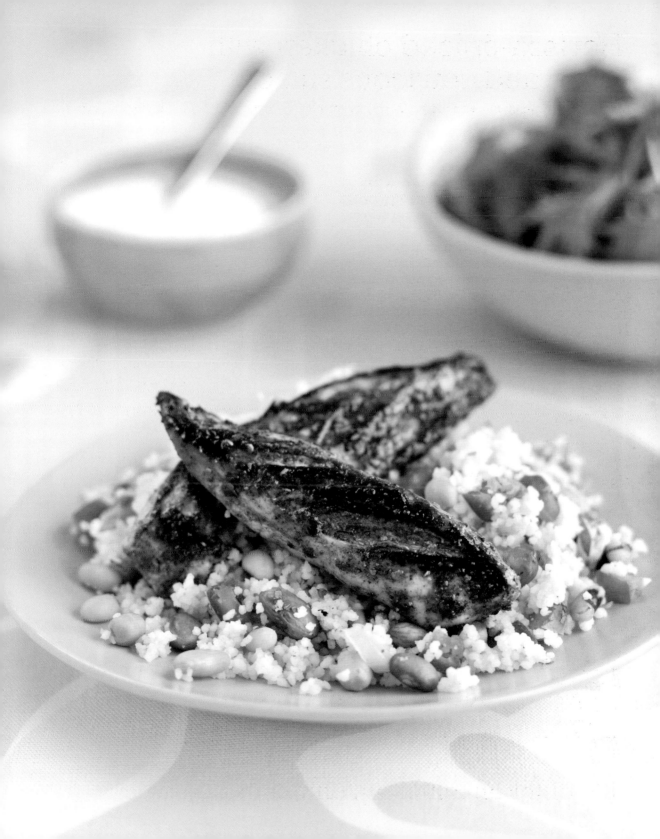

Mexican turkey tacos

Yes, it's turkey not chicken (you can use chicken if you want – minced turkey is easier to find), but these tacos are bursting with quick and simple Mexican flavours without all the calories. Turkey is a fantastically lean meat, and these zingy tacos will quickly become a family favourite!

serves 6
prep time 10 minutes
cooking time 35 minutes
362 calories per serving

500g minced turkey
1 small red onion
extra-virgin olive oil spray
1 pack (35g) taco seasoning mix
1 × 400g tin tomatoes
1 × 400g tin red kidney beans in chilli sauce
50g green pepper, deseeded and chopped
100g closed-cup mushrooms, wiped and sliced
6 taco shells
150g fat-reduced mature cheese, grated
a pinch of chilli powder
2 tablespoons chopped coriander

Preheat the oven to 180°C/fan 160°C.
Brown the turkey mince and onion in a large non-stick frying pan with three spritzes of the oil until the onion is soft. Stir in the taco mix. Add the tomatoes, kidney beans, pepper, mushrooms and a little water, and simmer for 15 minutes.
Transfer into a large casserole dish. Snap the taco shells in half, and arrange them to cover the turkey mixture. Top with the cheese and a sprinkling of chilli powder.
Bake in the oven for about 20 minutes, until the cheese is golden.
Scatter the coriander over the tacos, and serve with salad and a blob of 0% fat Greek yoghurt (15 calories).

Chicken and mushroom curry

A quick, filling dinner. No one seems to notice that it's healthy, which makes it even better!

serves 2
prep time 40 minutes
cooking time 30 minutes
179 calories per serving
359 calories per serving with 50g raw rice per portion

2 × 100g skinless free-range chicken breasts
vegetable oil spray
500g closed-cup mushrooms, wiped and quartered
1 large chilli, deseeded and finely chopped
2 cloves of garlic, chopped
6 spring onions, roughly chopped
150ml chicken stock
1 tablespoon curry powder
1 teaspoon ground cumin
1 teaspoon ground coriander
salt and freshly ground black pepper
1 tablespoon 0% fat Greek natural yoghurt
fresh coriander, to garnish

Brown the chicken breasts slowly in a spritz of the vegetable oil spray.
Add the mushrooms, chilli, garlic and spring onions with 1 tablespoon of
water. Cover and bring to a simmer over a low heat, stirring occasionally.
Pour in the chicken stock, curry powder, cumin and coriander and
simmer, uncovered, for 20 minutes.
Add more curry powder or cumin if desired and salt and black pepper
to taste. Serve with boiled rice (see the tip on page 93 to learn how to
cook perfect rice), yoghurt and a sprinkle of coriander.

Chicken and mushroom risotto

This is an easy recipe that is deliciously filling and satisfying. Risotto is an elegant comfort food, and it makes a fantastic choice if you want to cook something impressive for a dinner party, or for someone special!

serves 2
prep time 10 minutes
cooking time 25 minutes
495 calories per serving

extra-virgin olive oil spray
1 red onion, finely chopped
260g skinless free-range chicken breasts, cubed
1 courgette, finely chopped
200g assorted mushrooms, sliced
800ml chicken stock
100g Arborio rice

60ml medium white wine
1 teaspoon salt
2 teaspoons freshly ground black pepper
1 tablespoon parsley, finely chopped
1 tablespoon low-fat crème fraîche
30g Parmesan, grated

tip

If you are not sure if you have got the risotto consistency correct, spoon a little onto a plate or bowl and shake it lightly from side to side. It should spread out slowly and gently. If it just stands still, it is too solid and dry, so add a little more stock or water. If a puddle of liquid forms around the spoonful of risotto, then it has too much liquid, so let the risotto sit for a while with the lid on until it has absorbed the excess liquid.

Spritz a deep frying pan or wok (preferably non-stick) with olive oil and cook the onion for 2 to 3 minutes until just soft. Add the chicken, courgettes and mushrooms, and sauté, stirring occasionally with a wooden spoon, for 10 minutes or until the vegetables are taking on colour and the chicken is cooked through. Add a splash of water if the chicken starts to stick to the pan.
Meanwhile, fill a saucepan with the stock and bring it to a gentle simmer.
Add the rice to the chicken pan and stir through to make sure it is coated with the chicken and vegetable juices. Fry for a further 2 minutes.
Add the wine to the chicken and rice, and stir until absorbed.
Pour a ladleful of stock into the chicken and rice pan and stir until it is absorbed. This first measure of stock will soak into the rice very quickly.
Add another ladleful and stir until absorbed again. Continue in this way until all the stock has been added to the rice.
Taste a teaspoon of the risotto. It should be al dente – soft on the outside, but with a slight bite in the middle.
If the rice is a little harder than you like, then continue to cook as before until it is to your satisfaction, adding a little warm water to keep the consistency like that of a creamy rice pudding.
Add the parsley, crème fraîche, Parmesan, and seasoning and stir.
Serve immediately with a fresh green salad.

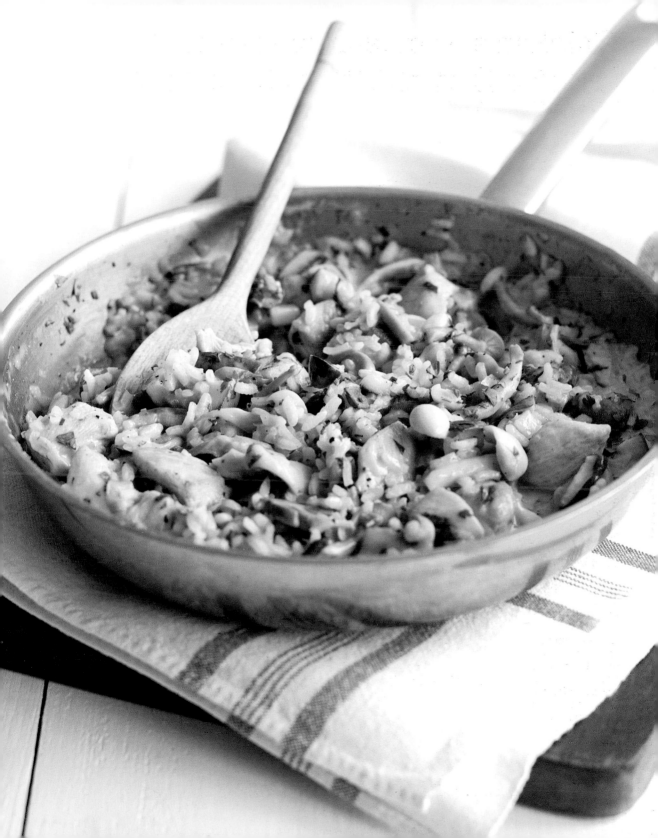

Jerked chicken with fresh mango salsa

A real Jamaican favourite, you'll find a 'higgler lady' on every street corner selling jerked chicken. Here's a quick and easy way to recapture that taste without using your air miles! Try using pork or prawns instead of chicken.

serves 2
prep time 15 minutes
cooking time 15 minutes
166 calories per serving

2 × 100g skinless free-range chicken breasts
1–2 teaspoons jerk marinade, depending how hot you like it (we like Walkerswood marinade, which is available in most supermarkets)
a squeeze of lemon juice
½ teaspoon vegetable oil
1 ripe mango (Alphonse mangoes are sweet and juicy and work well here), peeled and diced
1 tablespoon coriander, chopped
1 tablespoon lime juice
½ sweet red onion, peeled and diced
1 red chilli, deseeded and chopped (optional)
a pinch of sea salt

Make a couple of diagonal slashes in the chicken breasts. Put them in a deep-sided dish.
Mix together the jerk marinade, the lemon juice and the vegetable oil and pour over the chicken, turning once so the chicken is well and truly coated. Leave for as long as you've got, even if it's only 10 minutes!
Mix together the mango, coriander, lime juice, red onion and the chilli, if using. Season with a pinch of sea salt.
Heat a griddle pan over a low hob. Place the chicken on the griddle pan and cook gently (you don't want it charred on the outside and raw in the middle). It should take between 7 to 10 minutes on each side, depending on the thickness of the chicken breasts, until they're cooked through and smelling heavenly.
Serve with the mango salsa.

tip
If you can't find a ripe, juicy mango, use peaches or nectarines as a substitute. You can also cook this on the barbecue.

Warm chicken liver and apple salad

Chicken livers are delicious, healthy, economical and full of iron and vitamins. This is a simple recipe that tastes really special.

serves 4
prep time 10 minutes
cooking time 15 minutes
135 calories per serving

olive oil spray
2 teaspoons unsalted butter
2 apples, preferably Cox's Orange Pippin, peeled, cored
    and each cut into eight pieces
400g chicken livers, thawed if frozen, and trimmed
2 tablespoons red wine or sherry vinegar
salt and pepper
4–6 fresh sage leaves, chopped
mixed leaves or lettuce of your choice

Spray a couple of spritzes of oil into a non-stick frying pan over a medium heat with the butter. Add the apple slices and sauté until they begin to soften – 2 to 3 minutes. Add the livers and sauté until they're cooked through – about 8 to 10 minutes.
Add the red wine vinegar and salt and pepper, and let it bubble up for a couple of minutes. Add the fresh sage leaves.
Spoon over a bed of lettuce and serve.

You can substitute any type of apple – this recipe is also great with grapes!

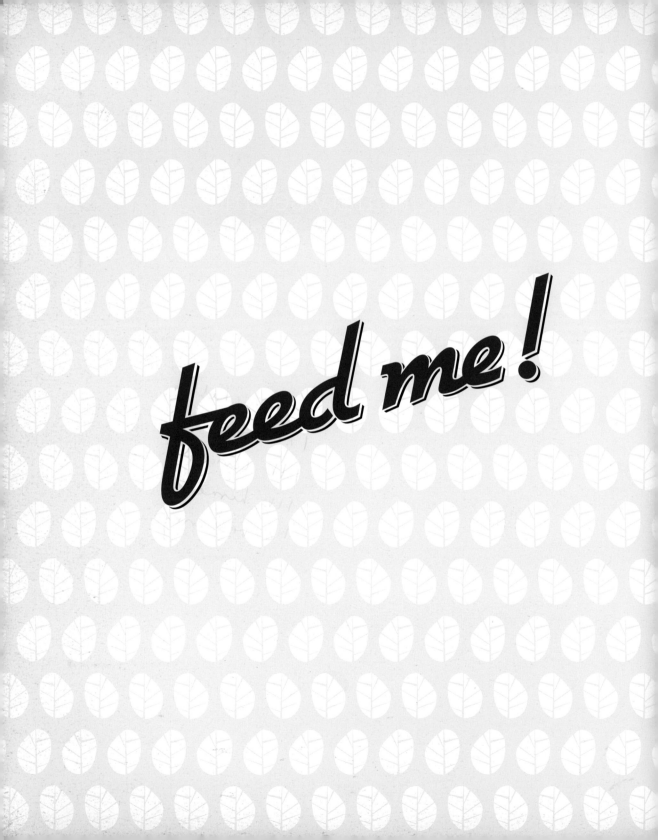

The ultimate fill-me-up dishes – but these ones are good for you! These are the recipes you need to turn to when you're absolutely starving and quantity seems just as important as quality. We've got a chilli, a hotpot, a risotto and a sausage pasta – proper, old-fashioned, rich comfort food that is as far from traditional diet meals as you can get!

Lamb hotpot

Although this recipe needs a long cooking time, it doesn't take long to put together and it's definitely worth the wait. A hotpot works really well for a family meal or dinner party because it doesn't feel like traditional diet food, so you don't have to make any excuses – you can just tuck in with the whole family, guilt-free. This is also a great way to pack vegetables into a meal without the children complaining. We like hotpot with mushy peas and mint sauce. Very Northern – very scrumptious!

serves 4–6
prep time 20 minutes
cooking time 1 hour 40 minutes
263 calories per serving (if serving 6)
395 calories per serving (if serving 4)

1 onion, chopped
1 leek, sliced
454g lean diced rump of lamb
light sunflower oil spray
1 teaspoon ground cumin
2 teaspoons chopped fresh mint
   or 1 teaspoon dried mint
2 tablespoons plain flour mixed
   with 2 tablespoons cold water

3 lamb stock cubes
200g carrots, sliced
100g Savoy cabbage, shredded
400g Charlotte potatoes, sliced
300g sweet potatoes, peeled
   and sliced
sea salt and freshly ground
   black pepper

Preheat the oven to 190°C/fan 170°C.
Sauté the onion, leek and lamb in a casserole dish with five to six sprays of oil for about 10 minutes until the meat is browned and the onion softened.
Stir the cumin, mint, flour mixture and stock cubes into the pan with the lamb. Pour boiled water over to cover and stir until the stock dissolves. Add the carrot and cabbage and stir. Put the lid on, and bake in the oven for 1 hour.
While the lamb is in the oven, parboil the sliced potatoes and sweet potato for 6 to 8 minutes, and set aside.
When the lamb has had an hour in the oven, arrange a layer of sliced sweet potato over the top of the casserole, and then a layer of Charlotte potato on top. Sprinkle with the sea salt and black pepper, and spritz five to six times with the oil. Put the hotpot back in the oven for 40 minutes without the lid, until the top is golden and crunchy.

tip

Freeze this hotpot in individual portions if you want an easy ready meal for those nights when you need instant nourishment.

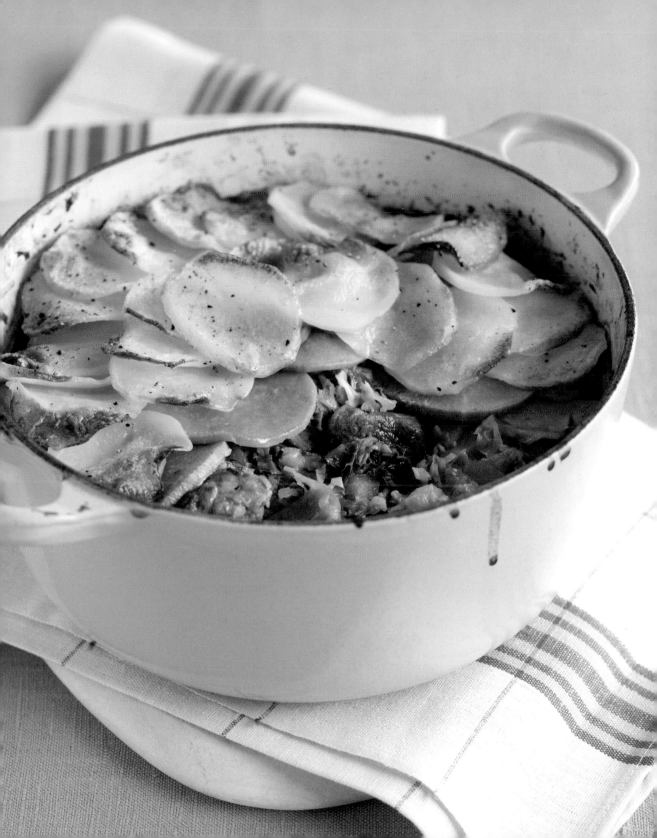

Panackelty

This is a reader's version of a traditional Northumbrian recipe. Her great-grandmother, a miner's wife, had 15 children, and passed the recipe down the family. Five generations later, the reader's children still enjoy their own great-great-grandmother's panackelty recipe as a warming winter dish. Cook this filling supper to start your own family tradition!

serves 4
prep time 15 minutes
cooking time 1 hour 30 minutes
352 calories per serving

340g premium corned beef, scraped of all the fat
300g onions
600g red potatoes
1 tablespoon olive oil
1 beef stock cube
5 tablespoons Worcestershire sauce
1 tablespoon fresh parsley, finely chopped

Preheat the oven to 180°C/fan 160°C.
Put the tin of corned beef into the fridge to chill the day before. This makes it much easier to cut thin slices (or just keep a tin in the fridge so there is always one ready).
Peel and finely slice the onions and potatoes. (Speed things up by using your food processor's slicing attachment.) Thinly slice the corned beef. Heat the oil in a frying pan, and sauté the onions for 3 to 4 minutes or until just soft. Blanch the potato slices in boiling water for 3 minutes, and drain well.
Make up a stock with 150ml boiling water and the stock cube. Mix the Worcestershire sauce into the stock (use less if you prefer a milder flavour). You won't need any extra seasoning.
Layer the onions in a 1¼-litre casserole dish with a lid. Layer the sliced corned beef over the onions, and finish with a layer of potato. Pour over the stock and put the lid on the dish. Bake in the oven at about for about 1 hour 30 minutes.
Remove the lid for the last 20 minutes of cooking time to make the top layer of potatoes go lovely and crispy. The potatoes and onions underneath should be completely soft.
Sprinkle the dish with parsley just before serving.

tip

Try adding layers of vegetables like carrot, parsnip or celariac. This is a very filling meal, and you may find that feeding six people with these quantities is more than enough!

Broad bean and bacon risotto

Risotto is a great dinner party dish – it's quick and easy, but still impresses. This recipe tastes creamy and luxurious even though it is low in calories. The dish is also very filling, so you won't be reaching for the snacks all evening! Great with a crunchy green salad.

serves 2
prep time 10 minutes
cooking time 25 minutes
461 calories per serving

150g broad beans, fresh or frozen
extra-virgin olive oil spray
1 onion, diced
4 rashers of smoked back bacon, trimmed of fat and diced
75g fine green beans, sliced
1 carrot, peeled and finely diced
500ml stock (use a cube if you don't have any home-made stock)
100g Arborio risotto rice
100ml dry white wine
20g Parmesan cheese, shaved
1 heaped tablespoon fresh herbs, chopped (most herbs can
    be used – we like a combination of flat-leaf parsley and basil)
salt and freshly ground black pepper

Boil the broad beans for 1 minute, remove from the heat and cool in iced water. Remove each bean from its thick skin and set aside.
Heat 10 sprays of oil in a heavy-based saucepan. Add the onion and cook gently until softened, around 5 minutes (add a little water if it begins to stick).
Add the bacon, green beans and carrot. Fry until the bacon is lightly browned.
Bring the stock to the boil in a saucepan.
Add the dry rice to the bacon mixture and stir thoroughly. Add the wine and stir for a minute, then add a ladle of hot stock. Stir until the stock is absorbed into the rice, then add another ladle. Repeat until you have run out of stock. The rice should be tender but retain a little bite.
Stir the broad beans through the risotto and continue to cook, stirring, for 1 minute.
Remove the pan from the heat and stir in the Parmesan and herbs. Season with salt and freshly ground pepper, bearing in mind the saltiness of the bacon and Parmesan. Serve immediately.

If you are in a hurry, you can add the broad beans without removing their skins. They will not be as tender, but they will still taste good.

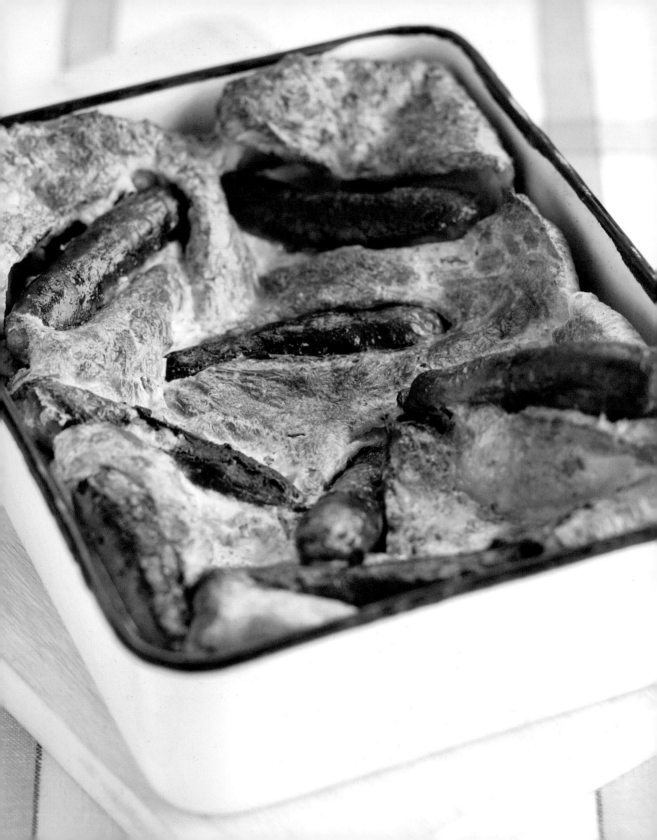

Tasty toad-in-the-hole with onion gravy

A healthier version of a classic. Reduce calories using skimmed milk and less fat – use these tricks to adapt other traditional recipes. A great alternative to a Sunday roast.

serves 4
prep time 15 minutes
cooking time 40 minutes
272 calories per portion

for the toad-in-the-hole
65g plain flour
100ml skimmed milk
1 medium egg
1 teaspoon rosemary
1 teaspoon thyme
1 level teaspoon salt
½ teaspoon ground black pepper
8 lean or low-fat pork chipolatas
1 tablespoon extra-virgin olive oil

for the gravy
1 teaspoon extra-virgin olive oil
1 large onion, cut in half and finely
   sliced
2 beef stock cubes
1 heaped tablespoon cornflour,
   mixed with 2 tablespoons
   cold water

Preheat the oven to 200°C/fan 180°C.
Sieve the flour into a large mixing bowl and make a well in the middle of the heap of flour. Pour the milk into the hollow you have created. Add the eggs and herbs, salt and pepper, and whisk, starting in the centre of the bowl and incorporating the flour from the sides until there are no lumps. Leave the mixture to rest at room temperature.
Prick the sausages and coat them in the olive oil. Place in a large (880ml) cooking dish and put into the oven for 15 minutes to brown.
Once the sausages have browned, pour the batter into the dish. Return the dish to the oven immediately and cook for a further 35 minutes, or until the batter has risen and is golden brown.
Make the gravy by frying off the onion and then dissolving the stock cubes and cornflour in 1 pint of water.
While the toad is cooking, cook any fresh vegetables you wish to serve with this dish and keep them warm. Retain the water the vegetables were cooked in for the gravy.
Fifteen minutes before the dish is ready, add the teaspoon of olive oil to a large saucepan and gently cook the onion until golden brown. Add 1 pint of the water the vegetables were cooked in to the onions, along with the stock cubes and cornflour mixture. Stir well and cook gently until thickened.
Cut the toad in the hole into quarters and serve with your choice of fresh vegetables. Spoon the onion gravy over the batter and enjoy.

It's important that any fat that has drained from the sausages during the cooking process is piping hot when adding batter to the dish. Do not open the oven door while the batter is cooking!

Quick marinades

A marinade can transform a piece of fish or meat into something really special at the cost of few calories. These are some delicious marinades for chicken, meat or fish. All will serve two, and are delicious for barbecues or grilling.

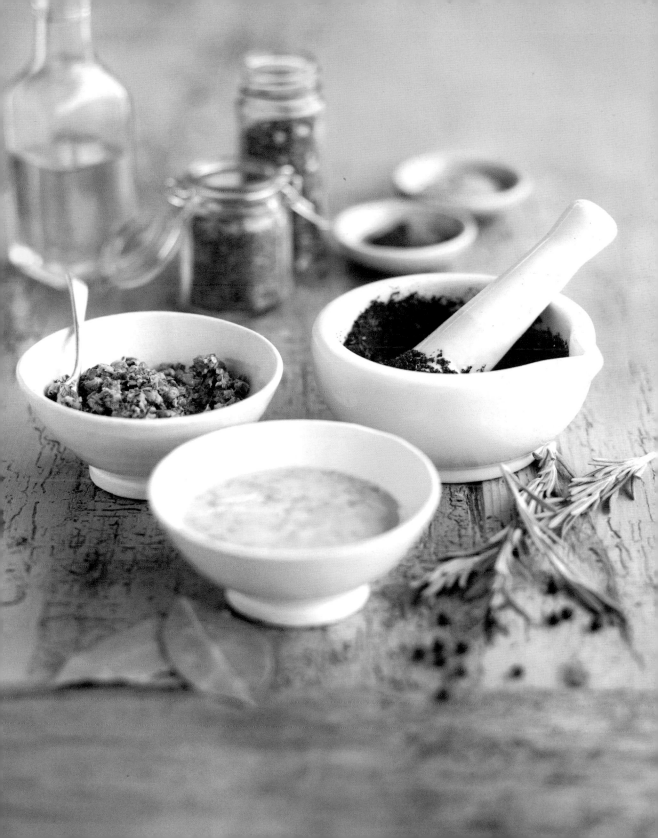

Quick beer marinade for steak

26 calories
2 tablespoons beer (leftover beer is ideal)
1 tablespoon Dijon mustard
1 teaspoon fresh marjoram
1 teaspoon crumbled dry bay leaf
freshly ground black pepper, to taste

Mix the ingredients together into a loose paste with a pestle and mortar, and smear all over steak before barbecuing or grilling.

Spicy marinade for chicken

23 calories
1 teaspoon ground paprika
1 teaspoon ground allspice
1 teaspoon ground coriander
1 teaspoon chilli flakes (adjust amount for your preferred heat)
1 teaspoon dried thyme
freshly ground black pepper
extra-virgin olive oil spray

Mix the dry ingredients together with the oil in a pestle and mortar. Rub well into chicken, turkey or pork. Leave, refrigerated, for as long as you can before grilling – this is delicious if you prepare it the night before you eat and marinate overnight.

A piquant marinade for fish

This marinade is ideal for tuna, swordfish or monkfish, all of which can take big flavours. We use lemon zest for a lemony flavour instead of lemon juice, because the acid in lemon juice would chemically 'cook' the fish. Not a bad thing, actually, but not what we want here.

13 calories
1 tablespoon chopped fresh rosemary
2 tablespoons capers, drained and chopped
finely grated zest of 1 lemon
freshly ground black pepper
extra-virgin olive oil spray

Mix the rosemary, capers, lemon zest and pepper into four spritzes of the oil. Rub well into your fish steaks and leave to one side until you're ready to cook.

There is no salt in any of these marinades. This is because the salt will slowly suck the juices out of the meat or fish rather than helping to add flavour. So make sure you season your marinated meat or fish with a little salt just before grilling.

Skinny lamb and spinach koftas

Adding spinach to this kebab mix replaces some of the calories from the lamb, and even improves the taste! As a wonderfully creamy alternative to the full-fat variety, we've used 0% fat Greek yoghurt. Good for everyday eating or entertaining – and only 188 calories per serving!

serves 6
prep time 10 minutes
cooking time 20 minutes
188 calories per serving
368 calories per serving with 50g raw rice per portion

90g baby leaf spinach
500g lean minced lamb
150g 0% fat Greek yoghurt
2 teaspoons ground cumin
1 teaspoon ground coriander
1 medium red chilli
2 teaspoons freshly grated ginger or 1 teaspoon ground ginger
2 × 400g tins chopped tomatoes
a pinch of salt and sugar, to taste

Preheat the oven to 175°C/fan 165°C.
Cook the spinach for 2 to 3 minutes (or just pop it in the microwave for 2 minutes). Drain, squeeze dry and finely chop.
Put the lamb in a large bowl, and add the yoghurt, the spinach, the cumin and coriander, half the chilli and a little salt.
Mix well, using your hands. Roll small balls of the mixture in your palms and place on a dry baking sheet (this makes about 36 balls). You can place them fairly close together because they will shrink in the oven.
Cook in the oven for about 15 minutes or until browned.
While the lamb is cooking, put the rest of the chilli and the ginger into a hot, dry frying pan and cook for a few minutes.
Add the tins of tomatoes, break up any whole tomatoes and stir well.
Add salt and sugar to taste.
When you have a nice thick sauce (this takes about 15 to 20 minutes), take out the lamb. It should be brown by now, but will have oozed lots of fat. Pour this away and mix the meatballs with the sauce.
Serve with boiled rice

These koftas freeze and reheat really well, so you can make double the quantity and put in the freezer in portions.

Quick lamb chops with a twist

Preserved lemons are a fantastic ingredient, especially with lamb. You can now buy them in most supermarkets and use them to add a delicious Middle-Eastern twist before grilling. You can even make your own – the simple recipe is in the tip on page 55. Serve this lamb with lots of greens, lightly steamed, and perhaps a small portion of couscous.

serves 4
prep time 5 minutes plus 20 minutes marinating
cooking time 8–12 minutes
276 calories per serving

for the marinade
1 tablespoon extra-virgin olive oil
1 small or ½ large preserved lemon, sliced
4–5 sprigs of fresh thyme
salt
for the lamb
4 × 100g extra-lean lamb chump chops, trimmed

Mix all the marinade ingredients, apart from the salt, together in a bowl. Add the lamb chops and rub the marinade into them well. Leave for as long as you have – if you 20 minutes, great; if you have an hour, better still. Even if you have only 5 minutes, it makes a difference!
Preheat a griddle pan to a medium temperature. Remove the lamb from the marinade, reserving the preserved lemon slices, shake off any excess oil (if you're doing these on the barbecue, the oil will drip off and catch fire), salt the chops on both sides and cook. They'll take about 4 minutes on each side for medium.
When the chops are cooked, set them aside on a warm plate to rest. Now take the preserved lemon slices and put them onto the grill pan. You want to have a couple of nice char lines on each side.
Serve the lamb with a crisp green salad and garnish with the preserved lemon slices.

tip
Remember that a great way to keep calories down and flavour up is to use herbs, spices and garlic – lots of flavour, very few calories!

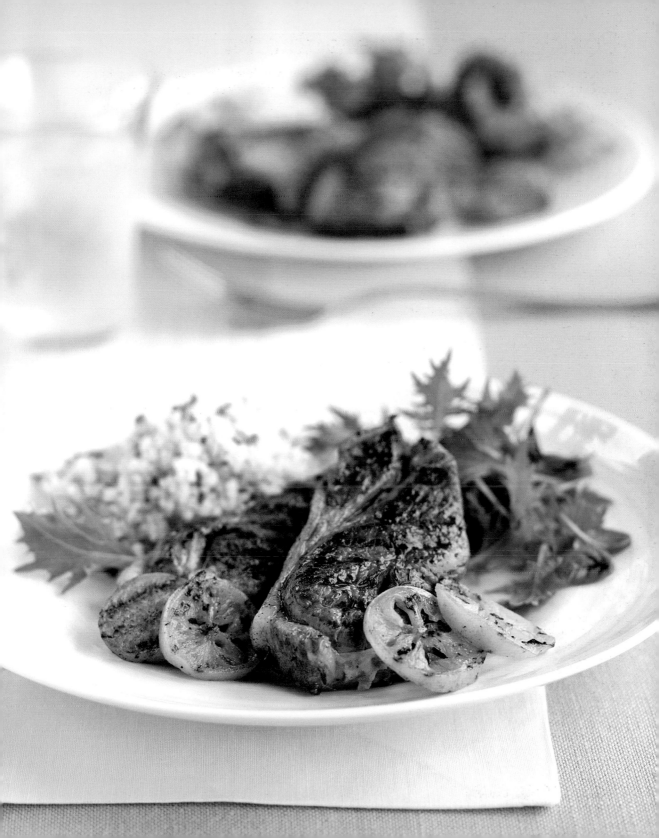

Pork chops with lemon and sage

Pork is a terrific and economical meat, and much lower in fat than you might think. Just make sure your chops are lean (you could substitute leg steaks for them, which are even leaner). This recipe gives an Italian twist with lemons and sage.

serves 4
prep time 5 minutes
cooking time 20 minutes
305 calories per serving

4 × 160g lean pork loin chops or steaks
salt and freshly ground black pepper
extra-virgin olive oil spray
juice of 2 lemons
6–8 sage leaves
1 tablespoon capers in white wine vinegar, rinsed and drained (optional)
1 teaspoon cold unsalted butter

Preheat the oven to 200°C/fan 180°C.
Season the chops on both sides with salt and pepper.
Spritz the olive oil in a roasting tray over a medium heat, and brown the chops all over.
Put the tray in the oven for about 15 minutes. Take the chops out of the tray and let them rest whilst you place it back on the heat.
Add the lemon juice, watch it bubble up, and add the sage leaves and capers (if you're using them). Season with salt and pepper to taste. Add the teaspoon of cold butter and whisk it in (this step is optional, but a tiny bit of butter at the end adds a real gloss to the finished dish, and lots of luscious flavour).
Serve the chops on a bed of greens – we love cavolo nero or cabbage – and pour the sauce over them. You could also serve a couple of new potatoes or some grilled polenta on the side.

Having a jar of capers in the store cupboard is an easy way of ringing the changes with all kinds of fish, pork, chicken or lamb dishes. And they're the slimmer's best friend – a tablespoon of capers only weighs in at 6 calories!

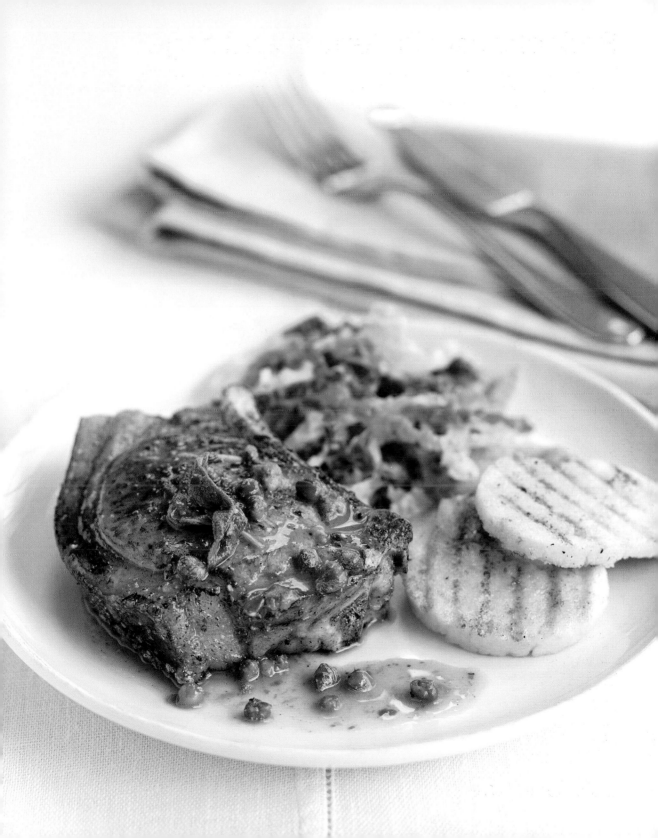

Linguine with sausage and cherry tomatoes

If you can find *luganica* sausage from the Lombardy region of northern Italy, do try it in this recipe. It's lightly spiced and mild, and (for a sausage), pretty lean. By and large, the Italians prefer to save their fattier sausages for stews.

serves 2
prep time 15 minutes
cooking time 20 minutes
415 calories per serving

150g pork sausages (preferably *luganica* sausages)
extra-virgin olive oil spray
1 clove of garlic, finely chopped
1 small mild red chilli, deseeded and chopped
8 cherry tomatoes
½ teaspoon chopped thyme
salt and pepper
100g linguine
1 tablespoon chopped parsley

Remove the sausagemeat from its casing and crumble into a bowl. In a heavy-bottomed, non-stick frying pan, brown the sausagemeat in a spritz of olive oil. As it begins to colour, add the garlic, chilli, whole tomatoes and thyme. Cook until the sausage is a lovely deep brown and the tomato skins have burst. Season with salt and pepper. Meanwhile, cook the linguine following the packet instructions. Drain the linguine. Pour it into a serving bowl and spritz the pasta quickly with olive oil. Add the parsley and the sausage sauce. Stir together well and serve with a green salad.

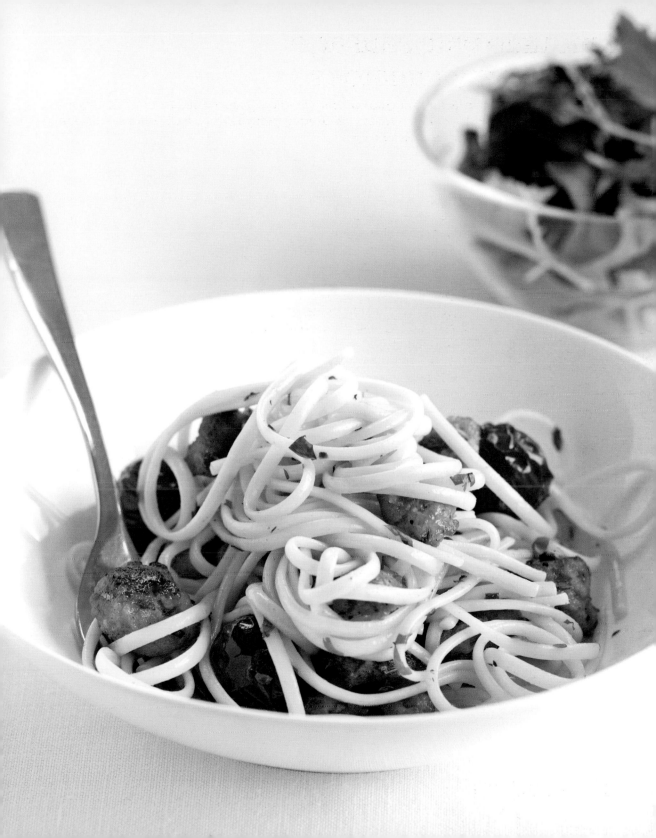

Sticky lamb kebab

We love this simple, tasty dish. It makes a really satisfying lunch just served on a bed of salad leaves, and is better than any take-away version we've ever tried!

serves 4
prep time 10 minutes
cooking time 30 minutes
233 calories per serving

1 onion, finely chopped
1 red pepper, finely chopped
100g butternut squash, finely chopped
454g diced lean lamb (such as leg steaks)
1 teaspoon dried mint
1 teaspoon ground cumin
olive oil spray
1 lamb stock cube
fresh baby leaf salad
½ pomegranate

Fry the onion, pepper and butternut squash over a gentle heat with the diced lamb, mint and cumin in six spritzes of oil for 6 to 8 minutes. Once gently browned, stir in the stock cube. You shouldn't have to add any liquid because the onion, pepper and squash will have released enough, but if it's very dry, add a tablespoon of water to help dissolve the cube.

Now, stir occasionally over a medium heat for about 10 minutes. It's ready when the squash is soft and any remaining liquid has reduced to a sticky coating for the lamb and vegetables.

Serve as it comes out of the pan on a bed of baby leaf salad with a sprinkling of fresh pomegranate seeds. For the ultimate kebab, serve in a wholemeal pitta with coleslaw. Phwoar!

tip

We sometimes make our own coleslaw to go with this using a bag of prepared crunchy salad tossed in a couple of tablespoons of light salad cream. It makes for a simple low-calorie coleslaw that complements this and many other dishes very well.

Beef shin and mushroom casserole

This is a very flavoursome, inexpensive beef casserole. We like shin of beef because if you cook it slowly for a long time, the meat becomes incredibly tender and the connective tissue just melts away, leaving a wonderful flavour. You won't find it in supermarkets, but any good butcher will have it – get him to prepare it in slices for you without the bone.

serves 7
prep time 20 minutes
cooking time 4 hours 30 minutes
224 calories per serving

14g dried shiitake mushrooms
9g dried porcini mushrooms
1kg trimmed beef shin, cut into
   2cm thick slices
14g sundried tomatoes
470g passata

1 bouquet garni
250g chestnut mushrooms, wiped
   and halved or quartered
2 teaspoons mushroom ketchup
   (optional)
10g cornflour

tip

The quantities may look huge, but if you have a casserole dish big enough, then you'll get loads of meals for the freezer. Like all casseroles, the flavour improves with time, so if you're organized enough, make the casserole the day before, pop it in the fridge when cool and just heat it up when you need it.

Pour boiling water over the dried mushrooms in a bowl. Leave for half an hour, then drain but keep the liquid. Preheat the oven to 150°C/fan 140°C. Dry-fry the beef slices in batches in the casserole dish just to brown them. While the beef browns, you can chop the dried mushrooms into thin strips, then cut the sundried tomatoes into tiny pieces (we use scissors). When the beef is all done, pour some of the mushroom liquid into the casserole dish and bring it to the boil, scraping all the lovely yummy bits off the bottom with a wooden spoon. Then layer the beef, chopped dried mushrooms, chopped sundried tomatoes and passata in the casserole dish and add a bouquet garni.

Pour over enough mushroom-soaking liquid to barely cover the meat. Bring it all to simmering point on the hob then place in the oven, covered. Leave for 3 hours, checking the level of the cooking liquid from time to time. If it is evaporating too quickly, add a little more stock. When the beef has been cooking for 3 hours, add the chestnut mushrooms to the casserole and give it all a good stir. The meat should be breaking into pieces. Cook for another ½ hour.

At the end of the cooking time, take the casserole out and taste it. If you want a more intense flavour, add the mushroom ketchup. Add salt if you feel it needs it. A little cornflour mixed with cold water will thicken the sauce. Don't forget to remove the bouquet garni before serving! Serve with boiled new potatoes or mash and a nice green veg or peas.

Barbecue time

When we do get a summer in the UK, a barbecue is one of the best ways to enjoy it. And if the weather's not behaving, don't despair – all these barbecue dishes can also be cooked on a griddle pan or under the conventional grill if it's bucketing outside!

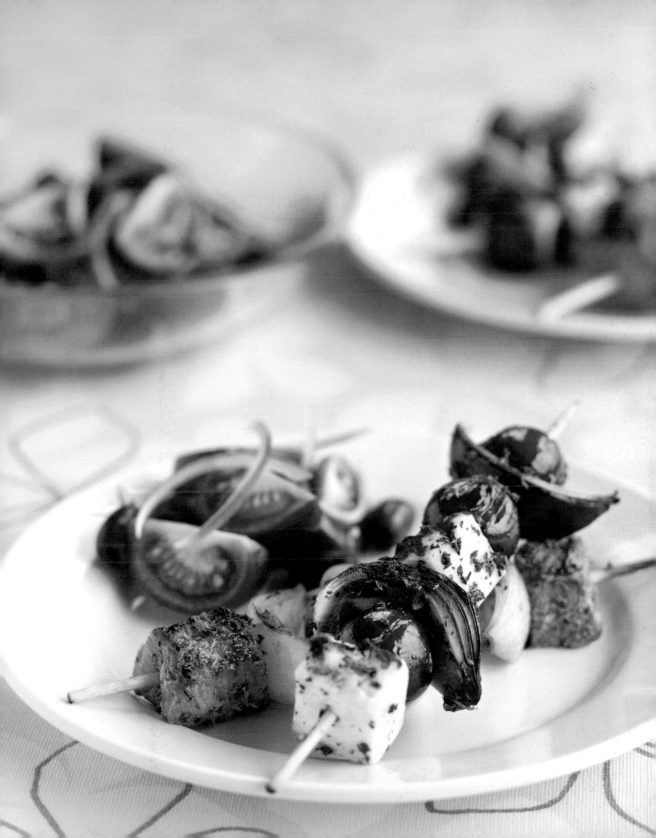

Quick porchetta

A classic Florentine dish.

serves 2
prep time 10 minutes
cooking time 10 minutes
170 calories per serving
2 × 100g pork loin chops, trimmed
2 teaspoons dried fennel seeds
2 teaspoons rosemary
2 teaspoons thyme
sea salt and freshly ground black pepper
½ tablespoon extra-virgin olive oil

Make 1cm deep slashes in the pork chops.
Mix the fennel seeds, rosemary and thyme,
salt and pepper and crush slightly to blend.
Add the olive oil to the herb mixture and
rub it well into the pork chops.
Leave for 10 minutes, covered, then cook
over medium coals for about 4 to 5 minutes
on each side until cooked through.
Serve with some grilled vegetables and
ready-made apple sauce, a squeeze of
lemon or, traditionally, in a roll!

Quick lemony Greek lamb kebabs

A dish for the Greek gods!

serves 2
prep time 10 minutes
cooking time 5 minutes
165 calories per serving
juice of ½ lemon
1 tablespoon dried oregano
salt and freshly ground black pepper
1 clove of garlic, crushed
olive oil spray

1 small onion
200g extra-lean lamb fillets, in 2cm cubes

Mix the lemon juice, oregano, a generous
amount of black pepper and the garlic
together with a spray or two of olive oil.
Coat the lamb cubes in the mixture and
leave to marinate for 10 minutes.
Peel the onion. Cut it into quarters and
separate it into pieces.
Thread the lamb cubes onto two skewers,
sandwiching a piece of onion between each
piece of meat. Baste once more in the
marinade, season with a little salt, and grill or
put over medium hot-coals for 4 to 6 minutes
until nicely charred and golden brown.
Serve with a tomato, onion and olive salad.

Halloumi and tomato kebabs

One for the vegetarians!

serves 2
prep time 10 minutes
cooking time 3–5 minutes
256 calories per serving
1 red onion
200g low-fat halloumi, cut in 2½–3cm cubes
4 cherry tomatoes or small tomatoes, halved
1 tablespoon dried basil
1 teaspoon dried oregano
freshly ground black pepper
extra-virgin olive oil spray

Peel and quarter the onion and separate it.
Thread the halloumi, tomato and onion pieces
onto two skewers, alternating ingredients.
Mix the herbs and pepper with a spray of
olive oil. Brush over the two kebabs.
Cook over medium coals for 3 to 5 minutes on
each side, until the halloumi is turning golden.

Texas chilli con carne

We love chilli; it's so versatile. You can have it on its own in a bowl with a nice salsa, with rice or on top of a baked spud. It keeps well in the fridge or freezer, and it's economical. This chilli is lovely served with the salsa cruda listed with the dips on page 217.

serves 4
prep time 15 minutes
cooking time 20 minutes
254 calories per serving
287 calories per serving with added crème fraiche

2 teaspoons vegetable oil
2 cloves of garlic, peeled and chopped
1 red onion, peeled and chopped
300g extra-lean minced beef
125ml red wine, stock or water
1 × 400g tin chopped tomatoes
2 teaspoons ground cumin
1½ teaspoons ground chilli powder (add more if you like it fiery)
1 teaspoon ground cinnamon
2 teaspoons dried oregano
1 × 400g tin red kidney beans, drained and rinsed
salt and pepper
2 tablespoons half-fat crème fraîche (optional)
1 tablespoon jalapeño peppers in brine, drained (optional)
1 tablespoon fresh coriander, chopped.

Heat the vegetable oil in a heavy-based saucepan and gently fry the garlic and onion until soft. Add the minced beef and brown all over. Add the red wine, stock or water and let it bubble up for a few minutes. Add the tinned tomatoes, ground cumin, chilli powder, cinnamon and oregano. Simmer gently for 10 minutes. Add the beans and simmer for another 10 minutes. Taste, and add salt and pepper accordingly. Serve with a dollop of the crème fraîche (if using), a few jalapeño peppers and a sprinkling of chopped coriander.

Try making a 'white chilli' by substituting turkey for the beef and cannellini beans for the red kidney beans. It's great with chunks of pork too.

Braised lamb shanks

Lamb shanks are delicious and economical, and make a rich, slow-cooked winter dinner. The great thing about this version is that you can make it well ahead of time, and then refrigerate or freeze until needed. To reheat, just place the defrosted lamb shanks in a preheated 200°C/fan 180°C oven for 30 minutes. This is a great dish when you are feeding family and friends. Try serving with plenty of seasonal greens and two or three egg-sized steamed new potatoes per person.

serves 4
prep time 10–15 minutes
cooking time 2¼ hours
323 calories per serving

2 teaspoons plain flour
sea salt and freshly ground
   black pepper
4 small, lean lamb shanks
extra-virgin olive oil spray
2 onions, sliced

2 cloves of garlic, crushed
750ml lamb or chicken stock
3 large carrots, chopped
1 tablespoon Dijon mustard
500g spinach, trimmed
a bunch of fresh basil

Season the flour with sea salt and freshly ground black pepper, then toss the lamb shanks in it so that they are lightly dusted. Shake off any excess flour.

Brown the lamb shanks thoroughly in a frying pan spritzed with olive oil. Once they are a golden brown on the outside, put them into a casserole dish.

Soften the onion and garlic in the frying pan, adding a little more oil if necessary. Once they are soft and translucent, add them to the casserole dish as well.

Deglaze the frying pan with a ladleful of the stock, scraping up the cooking residues. Pour it over the lamb.

Add the carrot, mustard and the rest of the stock to the casserole. Bring the casserole to the boil on the hob, then cover and simmer over a gentle heat for about 2 hours, stirring occasionally. Check there is enough liquid in the pan – if it is looking a little dry, add some water to keep it going.

Remove the lid and skim off any excess fat. Add the spinach and the basil and cook, stirring, until the leaves are wilted.

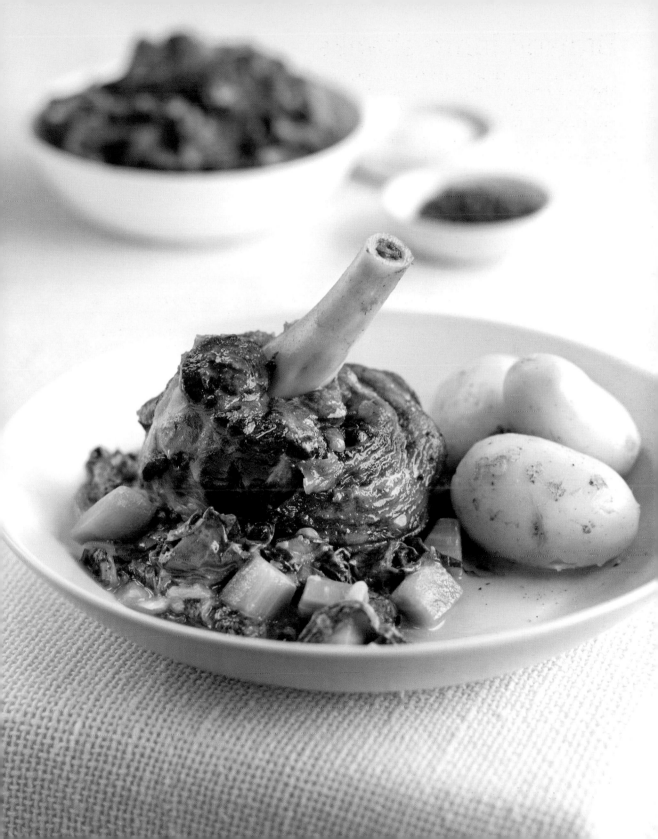

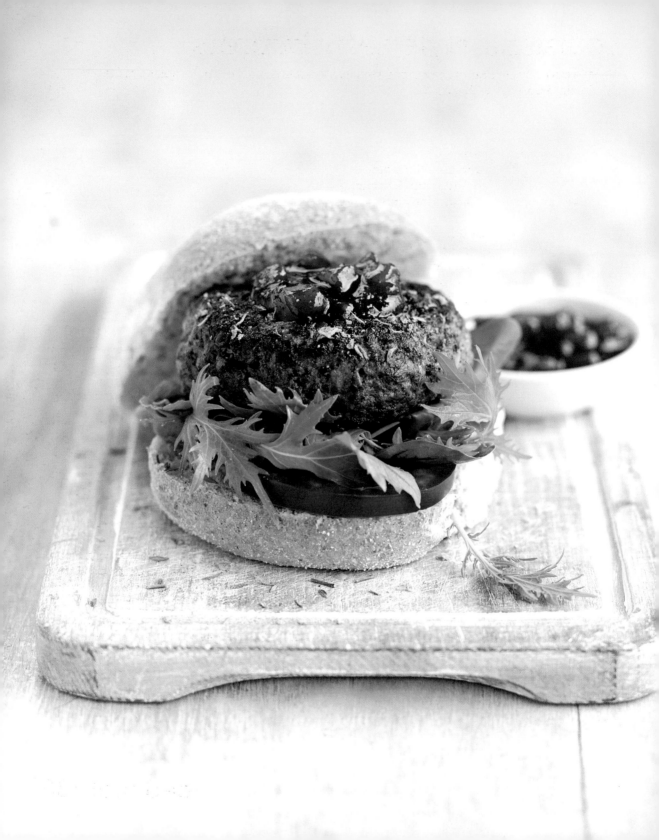

Louisiana-style zesty burgers

We love down-home Southern cooking with its spice and soul. Louisiana spices make a plain old burger go with a zing!

serves 2
prep time 5 minutes
cooking time 10 minutes
188 calories per serving

for the zesty seasoning
½ teaspoon sea salt
½ teaspoon ground black pepper
½ teaspoon thyme
½ teaspoon ground cayenne pepper
¼ nutmeg, freshly grated
for the burger
1 shallot
½ clove of garlic
½ tablespoon flat-leaf parsley roughly chopped
200g extra-lean minced beef
olive oil spray

Mix together the sea salt, black pepper, thyme, cayenne pepper and nutmeg. Set aside.

Chop the shallot and the garlic in a food processor, then add the flat-leaf parsley and give it a quick pulse to mix. Add the minced beef to the processor bowl and whiz it all together quickly. Season with ½ teaspoon of the zesty seasoning and pulse again.

Take the meat mixture out and form into four small or two large patties. Heat a griddle pan. Spritz the burgers with two or three sprays of oil on each side to prevent them sticking and put on the griddle for about 4 to 5 minutes on each side or until nicely chargrilled.

Serve with crisp salad, lots of juicy tomatoes and maybe a fruity chutney in a delicious wholemeal bun, and allow people to sprinkle the zesty seasoning on their own serving. Alternatively, you could serve the burgers on a bed of roasted vegetables.

Make up a batch of the zesty seasoning and keep it in a jar to add a kick to other meat and fish dishes.

Normandy pork fillet

Fillet of pork is fantastic – it has a delicate flavour and it is as lean as can be. This recipe combines it with the classic French combination of apples and cream, replacing full-on double cream with lighter, healthier crème fraîche.

serves 2
prep time 15 minutes
cooking time 30 minutes
249 calories per serving

vegetable oil spray
200g piece of pork fillet, cut into medallions or slices about
    1cm thick and flattened a little with a meat mallet
1 shallot, peeled and chopped
½ apple, peeled, cored and chopped
1 clove of garlic, peeled and crushed
125ml dry cider
2 tablespoons half-fat crème fraîche
salt and pepper

Heat a few spritzes of the oil in a non-stick frying pan. Fry the pork pieces on both sides until they are cooked through. You may need to do this in batches – don't overcrowd the pan.
Once the pork is cooked, set aside, then add the shallot and apple to the pan. Cook until golden. You may need another spritz of oil. Add the garlic. Cook until it smells fragrant and garlicky. Now add the cider. Bubble up hard for 2 to 3 minutes to cook the alcohol and reduce the liquid.
Turn down the heat and add the crème fraîche, stirring well. Now add the pork to the sauce, coating it well, and season.
Serve with fresh steamed green beans and some carrots.

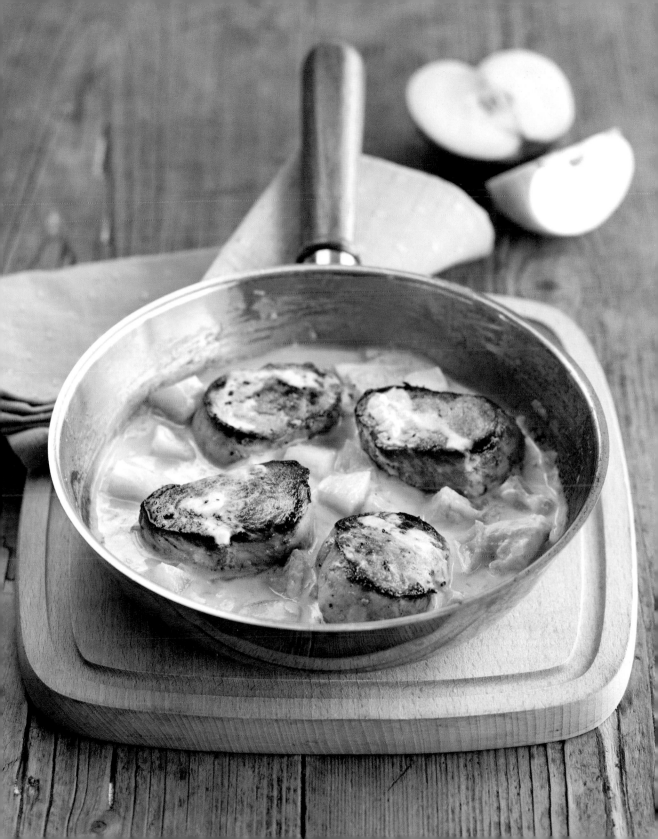

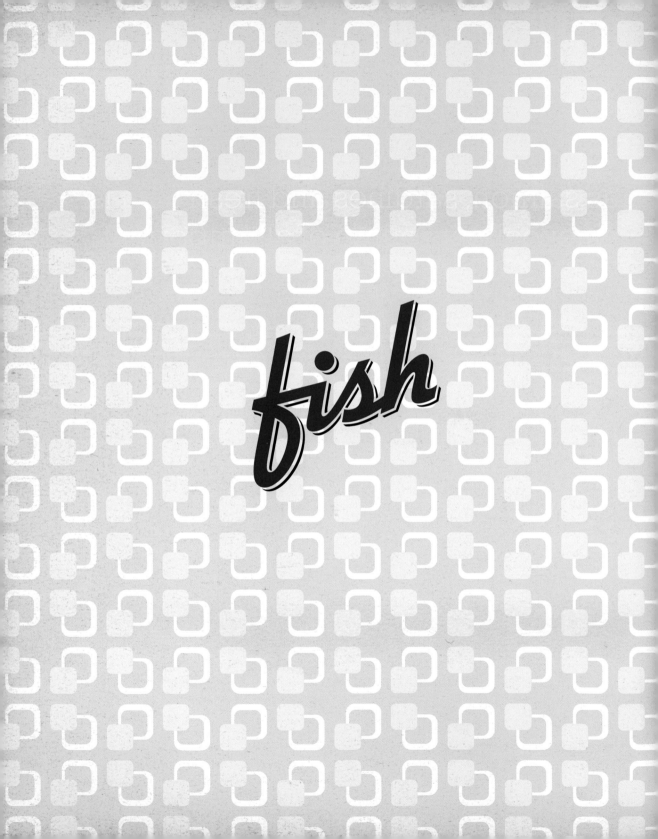

One of the best changes you can make to your diet is to include fish at least twice a week. White fish is low in fat and very low in calories, while oily fish such as salmon, sardines and fresh tuna is an excellent source of all-important omega-3 fatty acids. This is one group of fats that are actually good for us, and can help keep our hearts healthy. Using these delicious recipes, it is easy to include the official recommendation of at least one portion of oily fish a week.

Seafood lasagne

A great dish to share, this is a really tasty and healthy meal, which looks fantastic too. It does need some planning, but like all lasagnes, once put together, all you need to do is put it in the oven and relax!

serves 4
prep time 20 minutes
cooking time 45 minutes
502 calories per serving

30g butter
1 onion, finely chopped
40g plain flour
600ml skimmed milk
100g raw, shelled prawns
300g skinless cod fillet, cubed
300g skinless salmon fillet, cubed

juice of ½ lemon
salt and freshly ground black
    pepper
400g fresh spinach
3 sheets of fresh egg lasagne
    (not dried)
40g Parmesan cheese, grated

Preheat the oven to 200°C/fan 180°C.
Melt the butter in a saucepan and add the onion. Cook for 5 minutes over a medium heat until the onion is soft and translucent.
Stir in the flour and cook for a further minute. Gradually stir in the milk, a small amount at a time, over a medium heat. Make sure you stir continually as you add the milk until the mixture has begun to thicken and becomes a smooth white sauce.
Remove the sauce from the heat and add the fish and lemon juice. Mix well. Add salt and pepper to taste.
Wash the spinach and cook by covering with boiling water. Leave for a few minutes before draining very well.
Grease a 20 × 28cm ovenproof baking dish. Coat the bottom of the dish with about one third of the fish sauce.
Next, add a layer of the drained spinach, followed by a layer of lasagne strips, making sure the lasagne strips do not overlap.
Repeat the layering two more times, finishing with a layer of the fish sauce.
Sprinkle with grated Parmesan and bake for about 45 minutes or until the top is golden brown and the lasagne is bubbling. Serve immediately with a large mixed salad.

You can use 700g of any mixed fish, such as smoked haddock or cod. Try using a hand whisk to stir in the milk when making the sauce to ensure a smooth consistency.

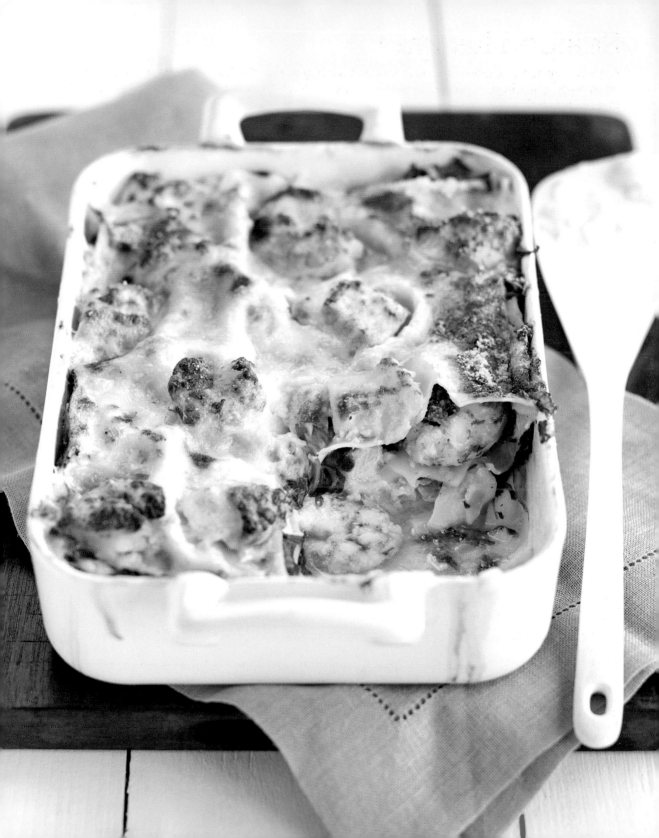

Spicy Italian coley

This dish is quick and easy to make. It's also delicious, with a great kick from the chilli. Made with simple ingredients, many of which you'll already have in your kitchen, it's a simple and healthy dish with plenty of vegetables to help you get your five-a-day. A spicy twist on classic Italian cooking!

serves 4
prep time 15 minutes
cooking time 30 minutes
364 calories per serving

2 small carrots, chopped into large chunks
2 stalks of celery, chopped into large chunks
1 small onion, chopped into large chunks
2 teaspoons extra-virgin olive oil
1 tablespoon tomato purée
1 teaspoon mild or hot curry powder
1 teaspoon ground chilli powder
1 teaspoon dried oregano
2 cloves of garlic, peeled and finely chopped
2 × 400g tins chopped tomatoes
salt and pepper
4 × 160g frozen coley fish fillets
200g spaghetti
a small handful of fresh basil leaves

Whiz the carrots, celery and onion in a food processor and blend until they are finely chopped.
Heat the olive oil in a large pan. Add the carrot, celery and onion and cook over a medium heat for 2 minutes to soften.
Add the tomato purée with the curry powder, chilli powder, dried oregano and garlic. Cook for another 3 minutes, stirring gently. Stir in the tinned tomatoes and bring to a gentle simmer. Add salt and pepper to the sauce to taste.
Add the frozen fish fillets, ensuring they are covered by the sauce. Leave the mixture to simmer over a low heat for around 30 minutes, or until the fish is cooked.
Cook the spaghetti in salted water according to the packet instructions. Drain well before serving.
Place a large spoonful of spaghetti onto the middle of the plate to serve. Spoon over the sauce, ensuring you also spoon out one fish fillet per person.
Garnish with the fresh basil.

You can use any kind of white fish in this recipe. Try a few different kinds to see which is your favourite! Freshly chopped chillies can be added to make the sauce extra hot and spicy!

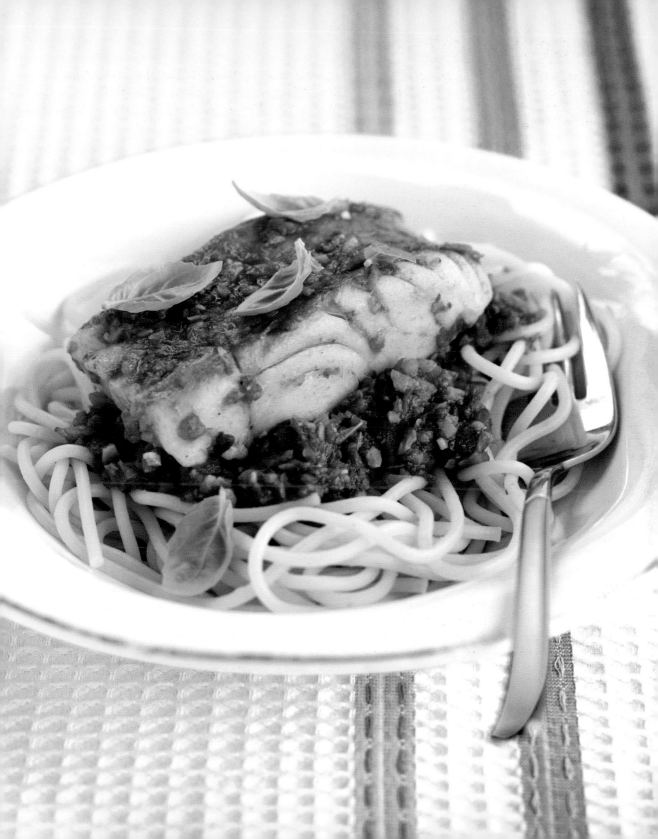

Oriental tuna stir-fry

This recipe is so quick and easy, and it's packed full of yummy goodness! Quickly stir-frying fresh vegetables over a high heat gives this dish a healthy, crunchy feel, and you can substitute any of the vegetables in the recipe for your own favourites. This is a great evening meal after a busy day, as you can have it prepared, cooked and on the table in no time.

serves 2
prep time 10 minutes
cooking time 7 minutes
282 calories per serving
462 calories per serving with 50g raw rice per portion

for the marinade
2 cloves of garlic, peeled and crushed or finely chopped
1 teaspoon grated fresh ginger
5 tablespoons soy sauce
2 tablespoons Chinese cooking wine or Japanese *mirin*
1 teaspoon honey
½ tablespoon sesame oil
for the stir-fry
200g tenderstem broccoli
1 large courgette, trimmed
1 bunch of spring onions, trimmed
250g fresh tuna, cut into bite-sized chunks

tip

We love to use Thai fragrant rice with this dish – try making it in the microwave so it's nice and sticky. Put ½ cup (90–100g) of rice in a microwavable bowl with a lid and pour over ½ cup cold water. Microwave and stir every 3 minutes until the rice is done to your liking. It usually takes 9 to 12 minutes in total.

Mix all the marinade ingredients in a large bowl.
Slice the tenderstem broccoli, the courgette and the spring onions into evenly sized pieces. Add them to the marinade with the tuna.
Stir all the ingredients well so that they are all covered with the marinade.
Heat a large wok or frying pan to a high heat. There is no need to add any oil. Empty all of the ingredients (including any marinade left at the bottom of the bowl) into the hot frying pan and stir-fry for around 7 minutes. You can stir-fry for less time (5 minutes) or more time (up to 10 minutes) depending on how soft you like your vegetables.
Serve on a warmed plate with boiled rice or see tip.

Spicy-sweet Thai noodles

This is a super-summery dish that will brighten up any day of the week. It combines crunchy vegetables with plump juicy prawns, all enrobed in a zingy fresh sauce that leaves you feeling totally satisfied. It's full of flavour, but not full of calories or fat. It's also really quick to make: this recipe will take you less than 20 minutes from start to finish.

serves 2
prep time 10 minutes
cooking time 10 minutes
472 calories per serving

1 teaspoon sunflower or vegetable oil
1cm piece of ginger, peeled and finely chopped
1 clove garlic, crushed
1 red chilli, deseeded and finely chopped
150g mange tout, trimmed
1 red pepper, deseeded and cut into bite-sized pieces
200g baby sweetcorn, cut diagonally
2 medium carrots, peeled and chopped into bite-sized pieces
2 nests (100g) of medium egg noodles
220g large cooked prawns, peeled
2 tablespoons sweet Thai chilli sauce
2 teaspoons cornflour
1 tablespoon light soy sauce

tip

For more zing, finish by adding some roughly chopped coriander and a squeeze of lime. For a change, you can also use chicken in this recipe, but you will need to add the meat to the wok and brown it before you add the vegetables. Otherwise follow the recipe as normal.

Add the sunflower oil to a medium-sized wok and heat over a high flame. Add the finely chopped ginger, the crushed garlic and the chilli. Stir-fry for 1 minute until the ginger and garlic release their aroma. Add all the prepared vegetables and continue to stir-fry for a further 3 to 4 minutes. Half-fill a large saucepan, bring to a simmer and add the noodles. After 1 minute of cooking, separate the noodles with a pair of forks and continue to cook for a further 3 minutes.

Put the prawns into a colander and rinse with cold water. Once the prawns are clean and fully drained, add them to the wok with the vegetables and stir-fry all together for a few minutes until they are warmed through.

Measure out 150ml cold water, the sweet chilli sauce, cornflour and soy sauce in a jug. Stir well and put to one side.

Once the noodles are cooked, drain and toss them into the wok and stir-fry until all the ingredients are fully mixed together. Now add the sweet chilli and water mixture while continuing to stir over the heat. The sauce mixture will start to thicken. When the sauce is thick, the noodles are ready. Serve in a nice deep bowl.

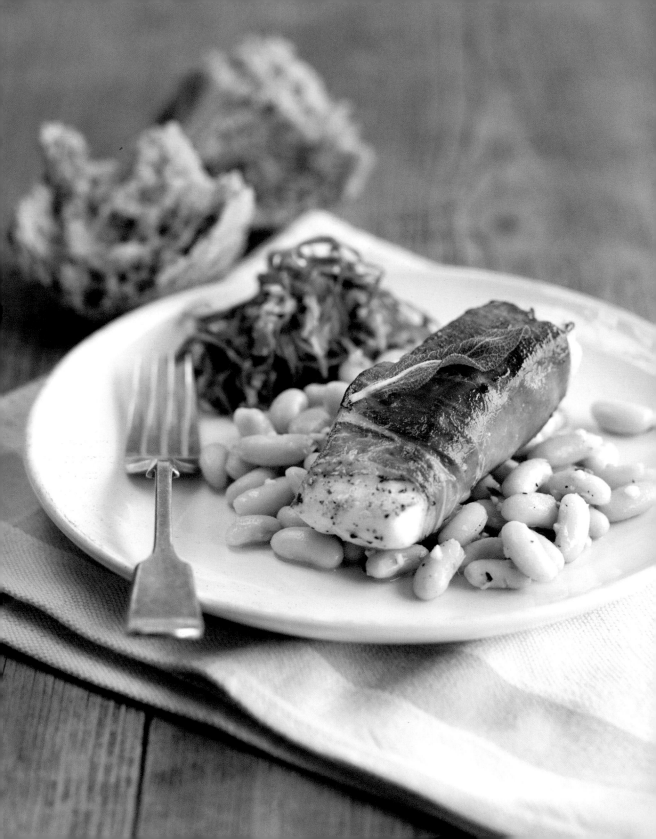

Cod saltimbocca

Saltimbocca is Italian for 'jumps in the mouth', and this combination of fish and prosciutto is full of lively flavours to wake up your tongue. Serve this on the bed of beans for fibre and add a green salad or some wilted lettuce. Yummy!

serves 2
prep time 5–10 minutes
cooking time 10 minutes
259 calories per serving

2 × 100g skinless pieces of cod
freshly ground black pepper
4 fresh sage leaves
2 lean slices of prosciutto
extra-virgin olive oil spray
4 cloves of garlic, finely chopped
2–3 anchovies, rinsed and chopped
1 tablespoon white wine
1 × 410g can of cannellini beans, drained and rinsed
a couple of sprigs of thyme

Dry the pieces of cod well, dust them with a grind of pepper and then place one sage leaf on each piece of fish. Wrap the prosciutto around the cod like a parcel, then place another sage leaf on top of the prosciutto. Heat a spritz of the olive oil spray in the pan and add the finely chopped garlic and the anchovies. Cook over a low heat until the anchovies have melted away and the garlic is soft. Add the white wine and the beans and heat through. Add some freshly ground black pepper and a sprig of fresh thyme, and set aside.

Put another spritz or two of olive oil in a wide, heavy-based pan and heat over a medium flame. Place the wrapped cod parcels into the oil and cook for about 5 minutes on each side – the prosciutto should be crispy and the cod moist.

Gently reheat the bean mixture and place the cod onto the beans on your plates. Serve with a side salad or some steamed greens and some crusty bread.

tip

Any good, firm white fish would work here. Get talking to your local fishmonger, and he can give you hints as to what works, what is in season and what is sustainable.

Simple moules

This is a cheap, easy and nutritious meal. Serve with a side salad or some crusty bread.

serves 2
prep time 10–15 minutes
cooking time 6–10 minutes
287 calories per serving

2kg live mussels in their shells
3 baby leeks, 1 large leek or
   1 onion, trimmed
2 sticks of celery
4 cloves of garlic
a large handful of flat-leaf parsley

2 teaspoons extra-virgin olive oil
salt and freshly ground black
   pepper
100ml dry white wine
200ml fish or vegetable stock

Put the mussels in a basin of cold water. Pick out any that don't close up when you tap them on the side of the sink and discard them – these mussels are already dead.

Scrape off any barnacles, using a little brush to clean the shells, and pull off the mussels' beards. These are the stringy, ropey, bits that the mussel uses to attach itself to rocks. Grasp the beard between your fingers and pull it sharply towards the hinge in the shell to remove it easily.

Chop the leeks or onion, the celery and the garlic as finely as possible. Then chop the flat-leaf parsley.

Heat the olive oil in a deep pot, large enough to hold all the mussels (make sure it has a good, tight-fitting lid). Now sauté the leek, celery and garlic over a gentle heat. As they begin to soften, add half of the flat-leaf parsley and some pepper.

Once all the vegetables are soft and fragrant, add the wine and stock. Turn up the heat and bring the liquid to a rolling boil.

Add the mussels to the pot and immediately put the lid on. Cook for 5 to 6 minutes or until the mussels are open. Give the mussels a good stir about half way through cooking so the ones at the bottom of the pot don't cook faster than the ones at the top.

Divide the mussels into serving bowls, then taste the cooking liquor. Season with salt to taste (you shouldn't need much) and add the rest of the parsley. Stir well, and pour over the mussels. Serve immediately!

If you are missing the garlic mayonnaise that traditionally goes with moules in Belgium, you can get a pot of low-fat thick yoghurt, add a clove or two of crushed garlic, a squirt of lemon juice and some salt and pepper, mix well, and dunk your bread in that!

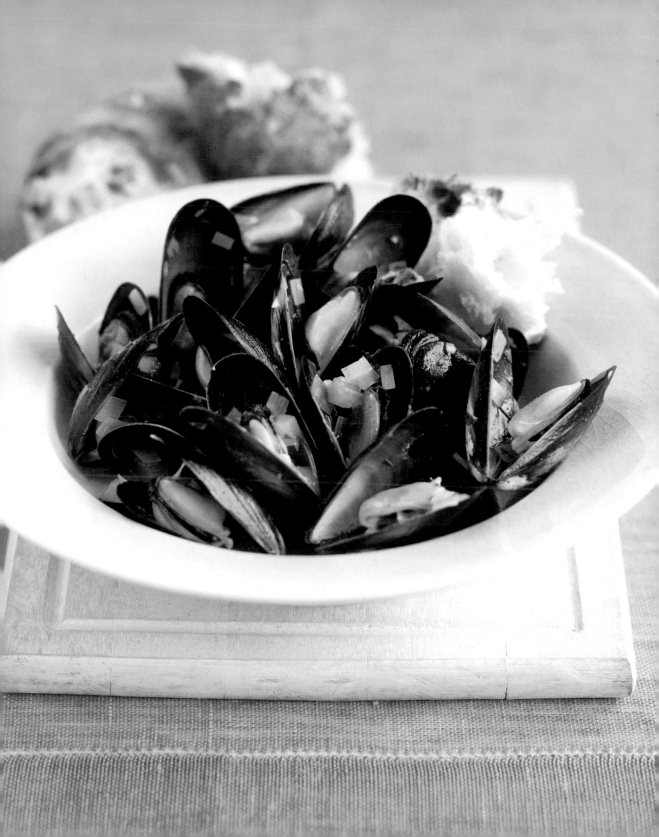

Steam-cooked salmon with soy sauce

This recipe has simple, healthy ingredients, and is fantastic for girly lunches and evenings when you don't feel like spending much time preparing dinner.

serves 4
prep time 20 minutes
cooking time 10–12 minutes
325 calories per serving

4 tablespoons light soy sauce
4 × 175g salmon steaks
3 spring onions, trimmed and sliced
3.5cm piece of ginger, peeled and finely chopped (you can grate it if you prefer)

Put 2 tablespoons of water and the soy sauce in a frying pan over a high heat.
Slide the fish steaks into the frying pan straight away, turning them once so that they are coated evenly with the sauce.
Scatter half of the spring onions and all the ginger over the fish.
As soon as the water starts boiling (this should only take about a minute), turn the heat down to low and put the lid on.
After 5 minutes, turn the fish and scatter the rest of the spring onion over it. Replace the lid for another 5 minutes.
Serve, spooning the sauce from the pan over the fish.
We like to serve this with steamed rice, watercress salad and a bowl of miso soup. You can buy miso soup in sachets – just add boiling water and garnish with chopped spring onions.

tip

To keep the salmon soft, juicy and succulent, do not cook the fish for any longer than 10 minutes. Use a non-stick frying pan.

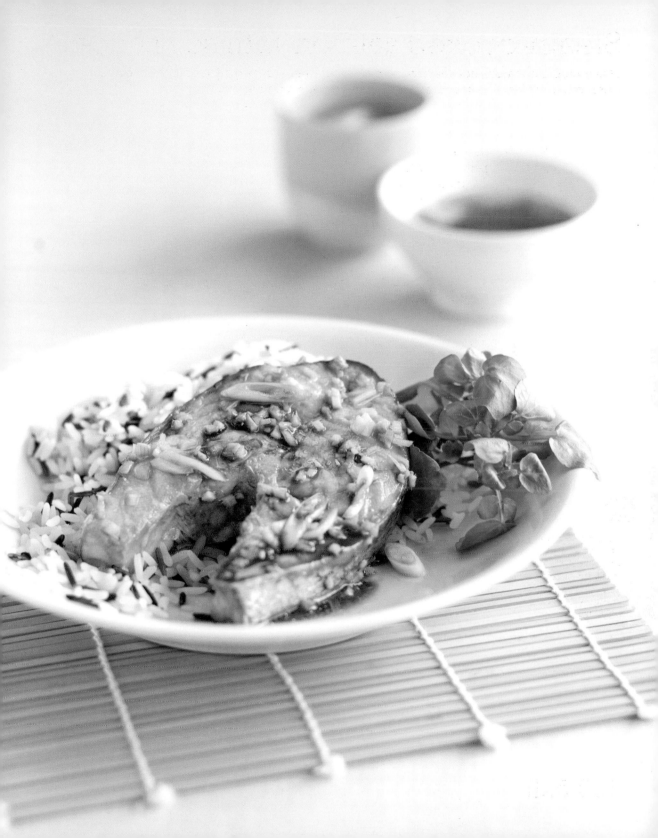

Seared ginger and soy tuna with vegetable noodles

This dish is so easy, and is as good to look at as it is to eat. You do have to plan a little in advance to get the tuna marinated, but the 5-minute cooking time definitely makes up for it. Perfect for a dinner party or romantic meal when you don't want to be rushed off your feet, this recipe has never failed to impress.

serves 2
prep time 10 minutes plus 3 hours marinating
cooking time 5 minutes
424 calories per serving

10g ginger, finely grated
2 cloves of garlic, finely grated
1 small red chilli, finely chopped
juice of ½ lime
4 tablespoons dark soy sauce
2 × 120–140g tuna steaks
salt

100g thin egg noodles
extra-virgin olive oil spray
1 red pepper, deseeded and
   thinly sliced
200g pak choi, sliced
½ teaspoon five-spice powder
2 teaspoons sweet Thai chilli sauce

Mix the grated ginger, garlic, half the red chilli, the lime juice and 2 tablespoons dark soy sauce in a small plastic food container. Add the tuna steaks and make sure they are covered with the marinade, pop the lid on and leave in the fridge for at least 3 hours.
About 20 minutes before you want to cook the tuna, remove it from the fridge.
Bring a pan of salted water to the boil and cook the noodles for 2 minutes. Drain and place to one side.
Heat up a large wok and, using a little olive oil spray, begin to cook the pepper, stirring constantly.
Slide the tuna steaks onto a hot griddle pan spritzed with some olive oil. Grill for 1 to 2 minutes each side.
While the tuna is cooking, add the pak choi and five-spice powder to your wok and stir-fry for another minute. Then add the noodles, the remaining 2 tablespoons soy sauce and sweet Thai chilli sauce and heat through.
Pile the noodles on two serving plates, and top each with a seared tuna steak. The perfect accompaniment to this dish is a mellow red wine – if your calorie allowance permits, of course!

tip

Use the zester on your grater to grate the ginger and garlic. This lets out all the delicious aroma and flavour, which will penetrate the tuna.

Paella fried rice

Quick, simple and delicious, this dish is perfect for an easy supper after a long day at work, or a lazy Saturday night in with the family.

serves 2–3
prep time 5 minutes
cooking time 10 minutes
378 calories per serving (if serving 2)
252 calories per serving (if serving 3)

extra-virgin olive oil spray
50g cured chorizo, diced
1 medium onion, finely chopped
1 clove of garlic, finely chopped
160g baby sweetcorn, sliced
½ red pepper, deseeded and thinly sliced
50g frozen peas
1 × 250g packet brown pre-cooked rice
125g cooked king prawns

If you like you can add a little chopped fresh chilli to spice this dish up, but it is good just as it is.

Spritz a wok with olive oil and heat over a medium flame. Add the chorizo, onion and garlic and fry for around 4 to 5 minutes. Turn the heat up. Add the sweetcorn, red pepper and peas. Continue to cook for another 2 minutes.
Add the rice straight from the packet with the prawns. Cook, stirring well, for a further 3 minutes. Serve immediately.

Smoked haddock and parsley fishcakes

A real comfort dish – just like mother used to make … almost!

serves 2
prep time 5 minutes
cooking time 35 minutes
133 calories per serving

175g smoked haddock (skinned weight)
100ml skimmed milk
5 whole black peppercorns
1 bay leaf
160g floury potatoes (we like King Edward), peeled and cubed
2 cornichons, drained and finely chopped (optional)
1 tablespoon finely chopped flat-leaf parsley
1 teaspoon plain flour
salt and pepper
vegetable oil spray

Skin the haddock if necessary and lay it in a shallow, wide pan. Cover with the milk and add the peppercorns and the bay leaf. Bring to a very low simmer – the liquid should be barely bubbling – for 5 minutes. Take off the heat and set aside.

Boil the potatoes and mash them, adding the chopped cornichons, if you're using them, the flat-leaf parsley and 1 to 2 tablespoons of the milk you used for poaching the fish.

Flake the fish into chunks, checking carefully for fine bones, and mix gently into the potato mixture.

Form into four patties. Lightly dust each one with a teaspoon of flour, (a tea strainer is perfect for this).

Lightly spritz a non-stick frying pan with four to five sprays of oil and heat over a medium heat.

Slide in the fishcakes and cook gently for 5 minutes on each side until nice and brown on the outside and hot all the way through.

Serve with plenty of peas and spinach.

tip

Try to buy line-caught and undyed smoked haddock if you can – you don't need any unnecessary artificial colours in your food.

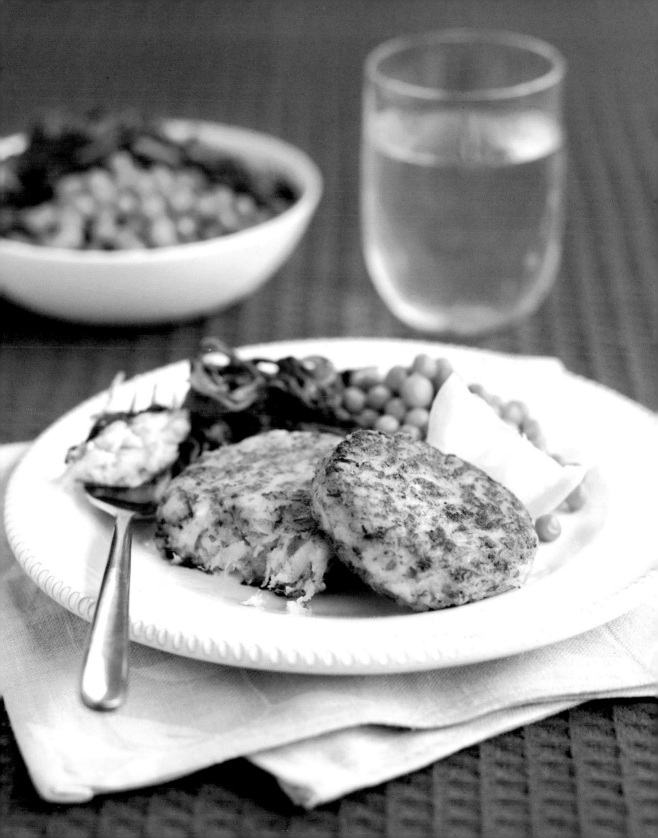

English trout cooked in paper

This is a classically simple summer supper dish for one, or for as many people as you want. All you have to do is make sure you have one trout parcel per diner. The great thing about trout is that it is always in season. It is also a low-cost, delicious and sustainable option for your omega-3 intake – and it's low in calories to boot!

serves 1
prep time 5 minutes
cooking time 12–18 minutes
303 calories per serving
483 calories per serving with 50g raw wild rice per portion

extra-virgin olive oil spray
1 carrot
½ bulb of fennel
1 × 375g fresh trout, cleaned
   and gutted

a small bunch of chervil
4 lemon slices
salt and pepper
1 tablespoon white wine
   or vermouth

Preheat the oven to 200°C/fan 180°C.
Cut out a piece of parchment paper and a piece of tinfoil to the same size as a baking tray. Lightly spritz the parchment paper with the olive oil and lay it on top of the tinfoil, oiled side upwards.
Slice the carrot and fennel into thin matchstick strips. Scatter them onto the parchment paper.
Wash and dry your trout. Lay it on top of the vegetables and stuff the chervil and lemon slices into its belly. Season with salt and pepper.
Bring the edges of the paper and foil up around the fish. This is the first step in making a parcel. Sprinkle the wine or vermouth over the fish.
Finish wrapping your parcel, carefully folding over the top two edges and twisting either end firmly to seal the fish inside a nice, airy shell with some room inside for the steam to expand.
Bake in the oven for 12 to 18 minutes or until the fish is steamed through.
Serve the parcel on the plate unopened. Then, when you rip it open with your knife and fork, you'll get to enjoy all the fragrant steam you've cooked the fish in and you'll have delicious cooking juices ready and waiting for you at the bottom of the parcel!
Serve with a 50g portion of wild rice (180 calories) or some boiled new potatoes, and something deliciously and seasonally green.

tip

Farmed British trout are easy to find and very sustainable, but if you can find a wild brown trout, so much the better – they taste delicious!

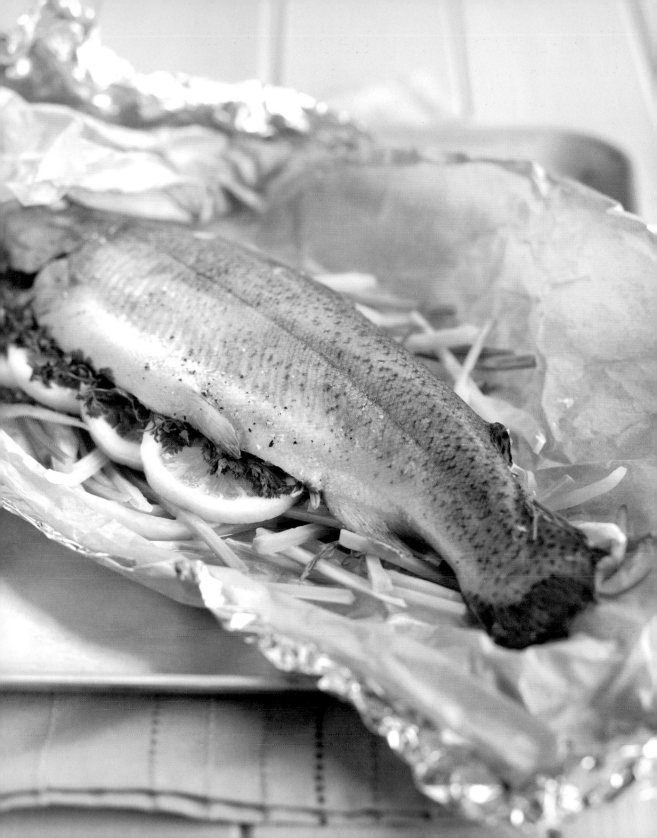

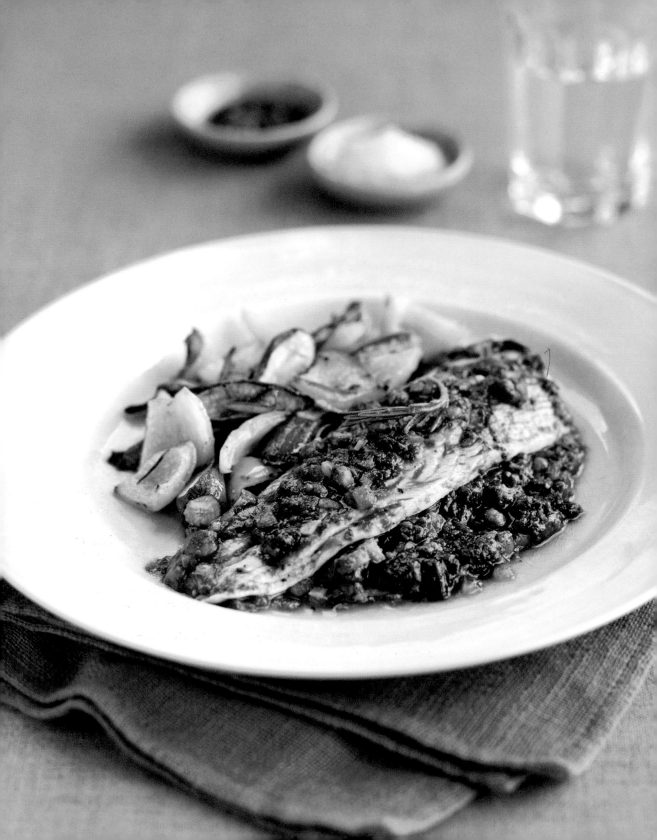

Sea bass fillets in a piquant tomato and rosemary sauce

This is based on a traditional Italian recipe for flat fish. With the added rosemary, this sauce is terrific with delicate sea bass.

serves 2
prep time under 10 minutes
cooking time 10–15 minutes
191 calories per serving

extra-virgin olive oil spray
½ onion, peeled and chopped
1 clove of garlic, peeled and chopped
1 × 400g tin chopped tomatoes
a small glass of white wine
1 tablespoon tomato purée
1 teaspoon dried basil
1 teaspoon dried oregano
a sprig of rosemary
1 tablespoon capers, rinsed and drained
2 × 80–90g sea bass fillets, skinned
salt and pepper

Preheat the oven to 220°C/fan 200°C.
Spray some olive oil into a saucepan. Soften the onion over a medium heat. When the onion starts to turn golden, add the garlic and keep cooking for 2 minutes.
Add the tomatoes, the wine, the tomato purée and the herbs. Bring to the boil. Add the capers, season and reduce the sauce until it's thick and delicious.
Spoon a layer of sauce onto an ovenproof dish. Layer the sea bass fillets on top and add enough sauce to cover. Bake in the oven for about 10 minutes.
Serve the fish on a bed of its sauce with some fresh green salad or roast veg on the side.

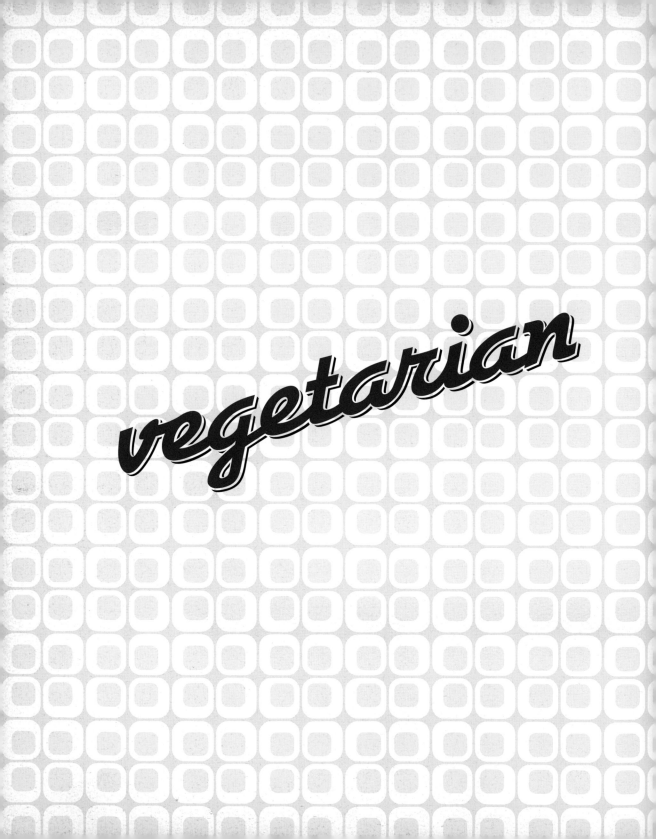

vegetarian

One of five important changes we talked about in the introduction was eating more fruit and vegetables. If you weren't sure how to do it, this chapter will give you all the help you need. All the world's healthiest diets, from the Mediterranean to Japan, are rich in vegetables. Bursting with flavour, fresh vegetables don't need lots of added fat, sugar or salt to make them truly delicious.

Garden-fresh quiche

This quiche is so fresh and full of healthy ingredients that even hungry teenage boys will enjoy it. (We know, because we tested it on one!) If you're running short of time, you could replace the home-made pastry with 250g ready-made shortcrust pastry.

serves 5
prep time 30 minutes
cooking time 25 minutes
286 calories per serving

50g hard, cold butter
100g plain flour
salt and pepper
6 asparagus
6 florets of tender stem broccoli
5 medium eggs
125ml semi-skimmed milk
60g mild soft goat's cheese, cut into small pieces

Preheat the oven to 200°C/fan 180°C.
First, make the pastry base. Use your fingertips to rub the cold butter into the flour with a pinch of salt, until you have a fine mixture that resembles breadcrumbs. Add just enough water to make the mixture come together and form a pastry, and roll out before the butter warms. The pastry should be cold enough not to need further chilling. Bake the pastry blind (with baking beans) for 10 minutes, remove the baking beans and cook for a further 5 to 8 minutes or until the pastry case is golden brown and crisp.
Steam the asparagus for 3 minutes and the broccoli florets for 2 minutes. Arrange the asparagus in the pastry case in an attractive pattern with the florets, cut into small pieces.
Mix the eggs with enough milk to provide a good depth of quiche, and pour into the pastry case. Add small pieces of goat's cheese where there is space, season, and cook in the oven for 20 to 25 minutes until the quiche has risen and the pastry case is golden at the edges.
Serve with a salad of new potatoes and tomatoes.

tip
Grate the butter to aid the quick mixing of it. Do not over-handle the dough – if your hands make it too hot, the pastry will not be as flaky and light.

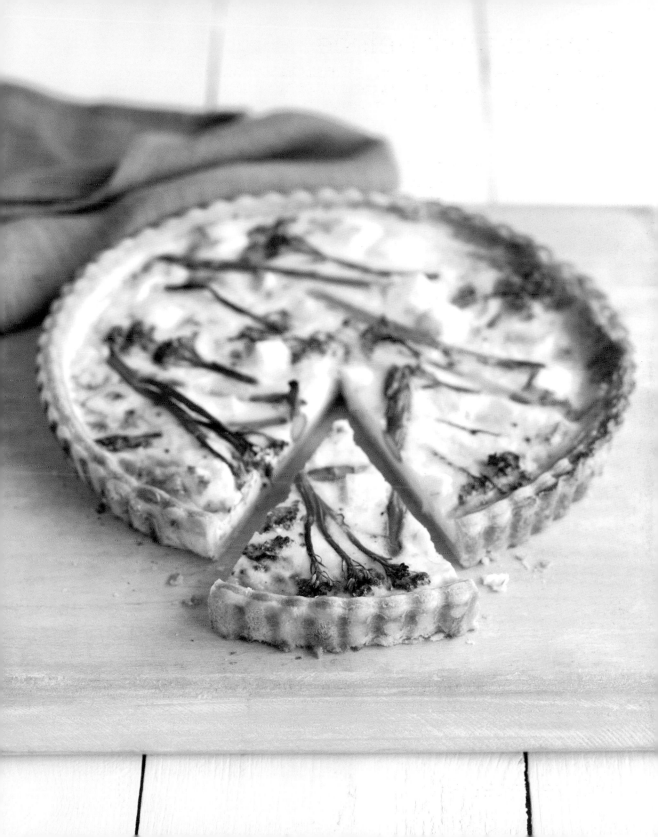

Spinach and cherry tomato frittata

Very easy and quick to make, this is a tasty, summery meal that is ideal with a large salad.

serves 4
prep time 10 minutes
cooking time 25 minutes
292 calories per serving

500g Charlotte potatoes
extra-virgin olive oil spray
2 medium onions, roughly chopped
110g fresh spinach, roughly chopped
75g cherry tomatoes, halved
salt and freshly ground black pepper
2 teaspoons Dijon mustard
6 large eggs, beaten
2 tablespoons grated Parmesan cheese

Cook the potatoes, still in their skins, in boiling salted water for 15 to 20 minutes until just tender.

Cut the potatoes into bite-sized chunks. Spray the pan with the olive oil and fry the onion for 10 minutes or until softened.

Heat the grill to a medium temperature. Add the spinach and potato to the pan so they are evenly spread over the base, arrange the tomatoes in the pan, then season.

Stir the mustard into the eggs, then pour the mixture over the top of the vegetables in the pan. Cook on the hob over a low heat for 6 to 10 minutes until the base is set.

Sprinkle the Parmesan over the frittata, then brown the top under the grill for 5 minutes. (If you are near your calorie limit, you can leave the Parmesan out and save 23 calories.)

Serve the frittata hot or cold with salad.

Luxury cauliflower and pasta cheese bake

A combination of two favourites in this dish lightens the calories, but doesn't compromise on any of the creamy, cheesy deliciousness that will be a hit with the whole family!

serves 6
prep time 10 minutes
cooking time 35–40 minutes
355 calories per serving

300g rigatoni pasta
800g large cauliflower, cut into florets
40g butter
40g plain flour
450ml semi-skimmed milk, warmed
1 teaspoon wholegrain mustard
60g extra-mature Cheddar cheese, grated

Preheat the oven to 200°C/fan 180°C.

Bring two saucepans of salted water to the boil and in cook the pasta according to pack instructions in one. Cook the cauliflower for 7 minutes in the other. When the pasta and cauliflower are done, drain them and lay them both in a large ovenproof gratin dish.

To make the sauce, melt the butter gently in a large saucepan. Add the flour to the pan and stir with a wooden spoon to quickly blend the two into a roux. Cook the roux for 1 to 2 minutes, then begin to add the milk and switch to a whisk. Pour the milk in, little by little at first, making sure you keep the mixture smooth and consistent. Once all the milk has been added, turn the heat up and bring the mix to a simmer. Change back to your wooden spoon and stir the mixture constantly.

Once the mixture begins to thicken, add the mustard. When it has thickened completely, add 45g grated cheese, reserving the rest for later, and let it melt into the sauce.

Pour the sauce over the pasta and cauliflower and mix it in. Sprinkle over the remaining cheese and bake in the oven, loosely covered with foil, for 25 to 30 minutes. Remove the foil 10 minutes before the end of cooking to allow the cheese to brown. Serve with a green salad.

tip

To tell if the sauce is done, coat the back of a spoon and run a line through it to see if your line will hold its shape. Buy the strongest Cheddar you can find to maximise on flavour for fewer calories.

Chickpea, spinach and cashew nut korma with pilaf

This is a fantastic vegetarian dish that takes no time at all to make and is absolutely delicious. You'll find this curry becoming a firm favourite, even with meat-eating friends!

serves 4
prep time 5–8 minutes
cooking time 20 minutes
499 calories per serving

for the rice
200g basmati rice
a pinch of salt
5 curry leaves
1 cinnamon stick
a pinch of saffron (optional)
for the curry
1 medium onion, finely
   chopped

1 rounded tablespoon
   korma curry paste
200ml reduced-fat or light
   coconut milk
1 × 410g tin chickpeas, drained
   and liquid reserved
200g washed and ready-to-use
   spinach
90g plain cashew nuts

Start the rice cooking first. The korma is done in the time it takes the rice to cook and stand.
Place all the rice ingredients in a pan and cover with enough water to come 1cm over the top of the rice. Bring to the boil and simmer, covered, for 8 minutes. Remove from the heat and leave covered until the korma sauce is ready. (Don't be tempted to take off the lid and have a peek until the curry is ready.)
Place the onion in a large, deep, non-stick frying pan with the liquid from the tin of chickpeas and bring to the boil. Lower the heat, cover and simmer for 5 minutes.
Remove the lid and gently cook for 2 to 3 minutes or until all the water has evaporated.
Add the curry paste and cook for 1 to 2 minutes to release the flavours. Stir in the coconut milk and bring to a simmer.
Add the chickpeas, spinach and cashew nuts and simmer for 5 to 10 minutes, uncovered, to heat through, wilt the spinach, combine the flavours and thicken the sauce. Season to taste.
Remove the cinnamon stick from the rice and fork through before serving with the curry. The rice looks pretty served in a tower mould. Serve with a fresh side salad or naan bread.

tip

Curry leaves are often available at Indian grocers'.

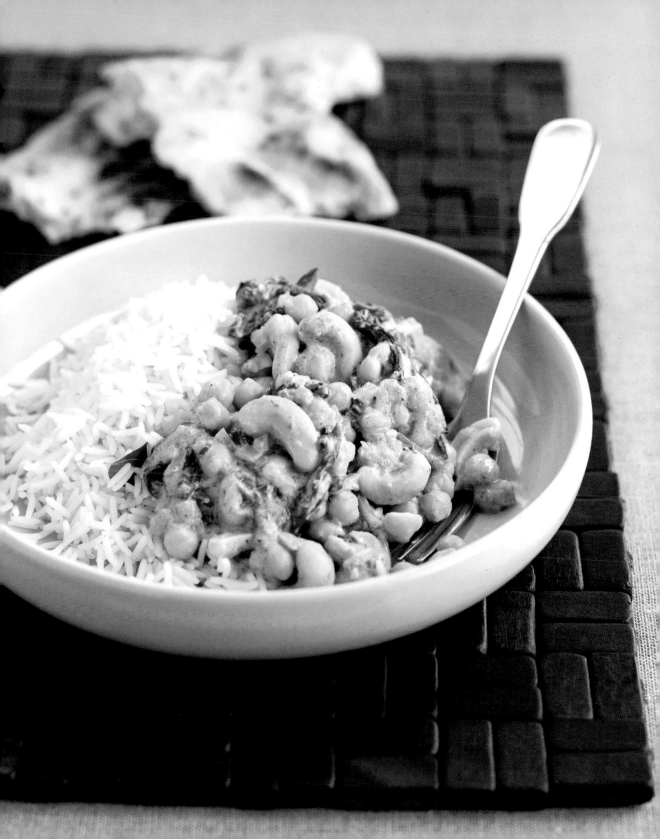

Jacket potatoes

A baked potato is such an easy, delicious and nutritious base for a variety of toppings, and cooking the perfect spud is easy. Floury potatoes, like a King Edward or Maris Piper, work best. A 180g potato is pretty much the ideal size. Preheat your oven to 220°C/fan 200°C. Wash the potato, but do not dry it completely. Roll it in a little sea salt, then pop it straight in the oven on the middle shelf for 45 minutes to 1 hour. When you take it out, your potato should have a crispy skin and a soft, fluffy interior. Listen carefully – it should sigh when you puncture it. Now, get topping! Each recipe makes enough to top one potato.

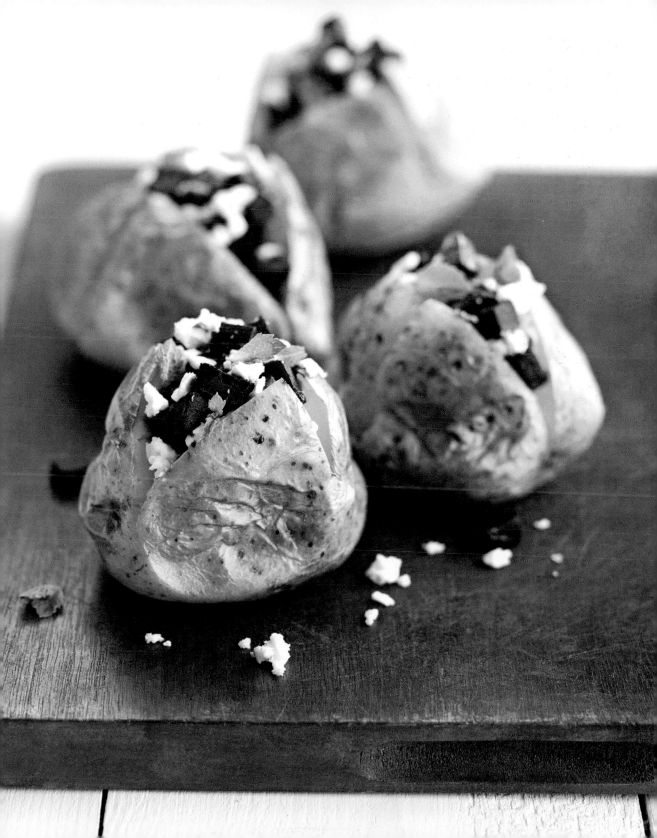

Tuna, spring onions, lemon, pepper and capers

Simple and classic, this is a sunny, Mediterranean potato topper.

79 calories per serving
324 calories per serving including a 180g baked potato

80g tin of tuna in spring water or brine, drained
1 teaspoon capers in white wine vinegar, drained well
1 teaspoon lemon juice
1 teaspoon extra-virgin olive oil
1 spring onion, trimmed and chopped
sea salt and freshly ground black pepper

Stir all the ingredients together in a bowl, and spoon into your potato.

Beetroot, mint and feta

Colourful and vibrant, sweet beetroot and salty feta cheese are a marriage made in heaven!

81 calories per serving
326 calories per serving including a 180g baked potato

25g reduced-fat feta cheese, crumbled
½ cooked beetroot, peeled and diced
½ tablespoon torn mint
1 teaspoon extra-virgin olive oil
1 teaspoon balsamic vinegar
salt and freshly ground black pepper
mixed leaves

Mix together the beetroot, mint, oil, vinegar and seasoning in a bowl. Cover and leave to marinate for 30 minutes to 1 hour while the potato cooks, then spoon into your steaming spud and crumble over the feta cheese

Tricolore

The colours of the Italian flag on a humble spud. Buonissimo!

171 calories per serving
416 calories per serving including a 180g baked potato

50g mozzarella cheese (try to get a proper *mozzarella di bufala*, which is made from buffalo milk, or use a reduced-fat mozzarella)
4 cherry tomatoes
1 teaspoon extra-virgin olive oil
sea salt and freshly ground black pepper
1 small red chilli, deseeded and sliced (optional)
a handful of torn basil
mixed salad leaves

Break the mozzarella into pieces. Halve the tomatoes and stir them together with the olive oil, salt, pepper and chilli, if you're using it. Shred the basil leaves into the mixture and stir again. Then spoon onto your opened baked potato and serve with the salad leaves.

There are several other recipes in the book which also make great toppings for a baked potato. If you have any leftover chilli, ratatouille, Provencal tian and so on, don't bin them – save them in the fridge for your next spud dinner. They'll all keep perfectly well for up to four days, and they all freeze beautifully too.

Sweet chilli tofu stir-fry

This recipe makes a quick, easy and tasty meal, and it's a good way to get a few of your five-a-day. It's simple to throw together when you're in a hurry, but want to eat something healthy. All the vegetable measurements can be 'give or take' when you're in a hurry. We love this vegan version because it doesn't sit on your tummy and is low in fat. Great for busy people on the go!

serves 2
prep time 5 minutes
cooking time 10 minutes
306 calories per serving
386 calories per serving with noodles

1 teaspoon sunflower oil
200g marinated tofu
5 tablespoons sweet Thai chilli sauce
1 pak choi cabbage, sliced into chunky strips
180g baby spinach leaves, torn in half
1 small red onion, sliced
100g bean sprouts
1 red pepper, deseeded and sliced
50g whole mange tout
5–10 baby sweetcorn cobs, sliced
½ head of broccoli, cut into bite-sized chunks
a splash of light soy sauce
100g wholemeal 'ready-to-wok' noodles (optional)
a dash of sesame oil

Heat the sunflower oil in a non-stick frying pan or wok until hot.
Add the tofu to the pan and brown on both sides.
Cover the tofu with the Thai sweet chilli sauce and stir.
Add the vegetables and a splash of soy sauce, and keep stirring for about 5 minutes.
At this point, add the noodles if using, and stir for 1 minute.
Stir in a dash of sesame oil.
Once the tofu is slightly browned and the vegetables are tender, serve in bowls with chopsticks – or you can cheat and use forks!

tip

Separate the noodles by giving them a squeeze in the packet before adding them to the pan to aid stirring.

Try serving the tofu over rice instead of using noodles.

Pastry-free chive and onion quiche

It's quiche, my friends, but not as we know it!

serves 2
prep time 6–8 minutes
cooking time 15–20 minutes
109 calories per serving
122 calories per serving with added onion

olive oil spray or a tiny knob of unsalted butter
½ onion, peeled and finely sliced (optional)
100ml semi-skimmed milk
2 medium eggs
a big pinch of freshly grated nutmeg
sea salt and freshly ground black pepper
1 tablespoon fresh chives or garlic chives, chopped
½ tablespoon grated Parmesan cheese

Preheat the oven to 200°C/fan 180°C.
Get out two 120ml ramekin dishes and spritz them lightly with oil
or a little butter.
Spritz a heavy pan with oil and sauté the onion if using. Take off the
heat and set aside.
Whisk the milk together with the eggs. Stir in the nutmeg and season
with salt and pepper. Stir in the onion, the fresh chives and the Parmesan.
Pour the mixture into the ramekins. Pop them in the oven for 20 to 25
minutes or until set and pale golden brown.
Serve piping hot in the ramekins with a nice, crisp green salad.

Try using different
vegetables –
blanched broccoli
and fennel, tomatoes
and red onions, red
pepper and chilli –
there are as many
variations as there
are vegetables. You
could also sauté
some garlic, replace
the nutmeg with
thyme or chervil –
there are a million
ways to customise
and make this dish
your own!

Dahl with okra and sweet potato

This isn't authentically Indian, but it's simple, quick and tastes delicious.

serves 4
prep time 10 minutes
cooking time 15 minutes
244 calories per serving
424 calories per serving with 50g raw rice per portion

1 teaspoon cumin seeds
1 teaspoon coriander seeds
vegetable oil spray
1 sweet potato, peeled and chopped into cubes
1 onion, chopped
3 cloves of garlic, chopped
300ml chicken or vegetable stock
300g okra, topped and tailed
2 × 400g tins of lentils in brine, drained and rinsed (210g drained weight)
1 teaspoon ground turmeric
1 teaspoon mild chilli powder (to taste)
¼ teaspoon chilli flakes
salt and pepper
100g feta cheese, cubed
1 tablespoon chopped coriander

Toast the cumin and coriander seeds in a dry frying pan over a low heat until they are fragrant – about 3 minutes. Set aside. Grind the spices coarsely in a pestle and mortar.

Heat 2 spritzes of the vegetable oil spray over a medium hob and fry the sweet potato, onion and the garlic until soft but not brown. Add the cumin and coriander and stir for another minute. Add the stock and bring to the boil.

Add the okra, lentils, turmeric, chilli powder and chilli flakes, and bring back to a simmer. Cover with a lid, reduce the heat and continue to simmer for 5 to 6 minutes. Add salt and pepper to taste.

Just before serving, add the cubed feta cheese and sprinkle with the chopped coriander. We like to serve this with a fragrant cardamom rice (see tip), but plain boiled rice is good too.

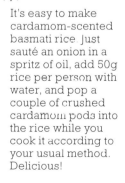

tip

It's easy to make cardamom-scented basmati rice. Just sauté an onion in a spritz of oil, add 50g rice per person with water, and pop a couple of crushed cardamom pods into the rice while you cook it according to your usual method. Delicious!

Provencal vegetable tian

The word *tian* just means a certain type of pot, used specifically for baking vegetables. It's narrower at the bottom than at the top, to maximise on the surface area for a bubbly-cheesy topping. This version cuts back a lot on the cheese to make it lighter, cleaner, and generally better for you. But it remains simple, delicious and very, very French. Bon appétit!

serves 2 as a main course or 4 as a side dish
prep time 10 minutes
cooking time 25–30 minutes
277 calories per serving as a main course
139 calories per serving as a side dish

extra-virgin olive oil spray
2 large onions, sliced
3 cloves of garlic, peeled and sliced
6 large tomatoes, sliced
6 courgettes, sliced
1 heaped teaspoon herbes de Provence
2 tablespoons fresh breadcrumbs
1 tablespoon grated Parmesan cheese
sea salt and freshly ground black pepper

Preheat the oven to 200°C/fan 180°C.
Spritz a non-stick frying pan with 3 sprays of olive oil, and sauté the onions and garlic until just soft.
Lightly oil an ovenproof gratin dish and arrange the onions and garlic evenly in the bottom.
Combine the tomatoes and courgettes in a bowl with a few spritzes of olive oil, the herbes de Provence and salt and pepper to taste.
Layer the tomatoes and courgettes on top of the onions and garlic.
Mix the Parmesan and the breadcrumbs and sprinkle over the tian.
Bake in the oven for 25 to 30 minutes.
Serve as a side dish or with a watercress salad as a main course.

tip

It's easy to make breadcrumbs – just drop slices of stale bread into the food processor and whiz.

174 vegetarian

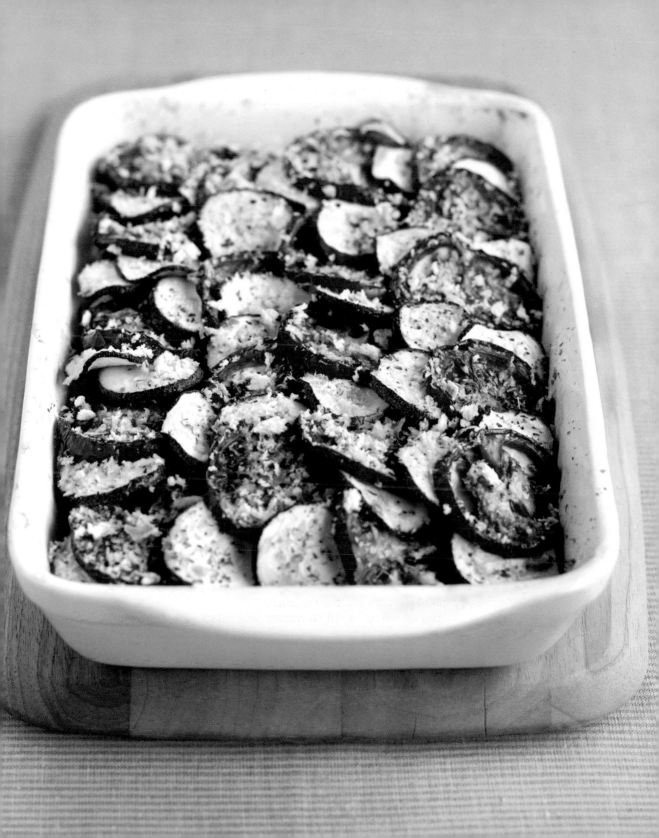

Roast asparagus on rocket with a Parmesan vinaigrette

Try this recipe when English asparagus is in season (May to June). Roasting asparagus capitalises on its natural sweetness. This makes a great light lunch on its own, perhaps with a slice of ham. It's also a lovely accompaniment to grilled fish and meat. As soon as asparagus is picked, its delicious sugars start to turn to starch, so go for local rather than imported when you can – it will be fresher, sweeter and more tender.

serves 2
prep time 5 minutes
cooking time 15 minutes
125 calories per serving

250g fresh asparagus
extra-virgin olive oil spray
salt and pepper
1½ tablespoons fresh lemon juice
1 tablespoon finely grated Parmesan cheese
1 tablespoon extra-virgin olive oil
200g rocket

Preheat the oven to 200°C/fan 180°C.
Trim the woody bits from the bottom of each stalk of asparagus. Spray the spears with the olive oil and lay in a roasting tin. Season with salt and pepper, and pop in the oven for about 15 minutes or just until they are cooked through and lightly browning in places.
Remove the asparagus from the oven and set aside.
Mix together the lemon juice, Parmesan and olive oil and salt and pepper to taste. Roll the asparagus in the dressing and place gently on top of the rocket.
You could also add a few cherry tomatoes or black olives.

tip

Asparagus also has a little trick up its sleeve. If you gently bend a spear at the bottom, it will 'snap' exactly where you need it to, right where the woody bit ends, so you can trim it easily. What a clever vegetable!

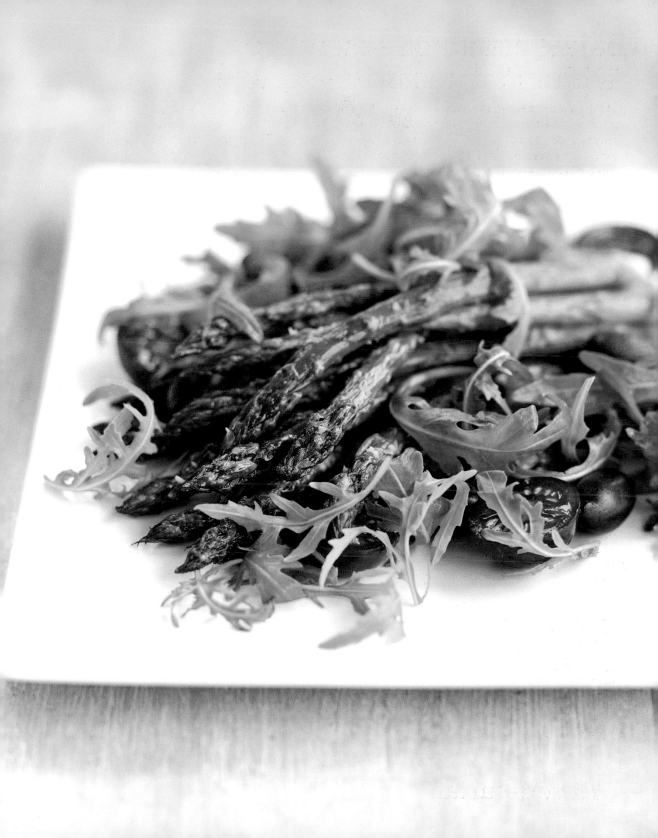

Baked goat's cheese and chicory salad

This is a really simple recipe for a sophisticated French lunch, with lots of bitter chicory to fill you up and excite your taste buds.

serves 6
prep time 5–8 minutes
cooking time 20–25 minutes
253 calories per serving

6 red or pale green chicory heads
3 logs of mild French goat's cheese with a rind
fresh herbs of your choice (we like a lot of thyme,
    but basil and flat-leaf parsley are good too)
extra-virgin olive oil spray

Preheat the oven to 200°C/fan 180°C.
Slice the chicory heads in two lengthways, then core them, removing the tough stalk and central core. Lay them end to end in a shallow ovenproof dish, or arrange two halves of chicory per person in individual dishes. Make sure the cut side is uppermost.
Slice each of the cheeses into four rounds and lay two on the chicory. Sprinkle with herbs and salt and pepper, and spritz each cheesy cut surface of chicory with extra-virgin olive oil.
Pop into the oven for about 20 to 25 minutes until the chicory is cooked through and melty, and the cheese is bubbling.
Serve with a salad of mixed greens on the side.

tip

Try using some different goat's cheeses. You can find ones covered in ash, wrapped in leaves or flavoured with herbs and wine. Do check the labels though, as goat's cheese can vary a lot in calories.

A nice substitute for the chicory is radicchio.

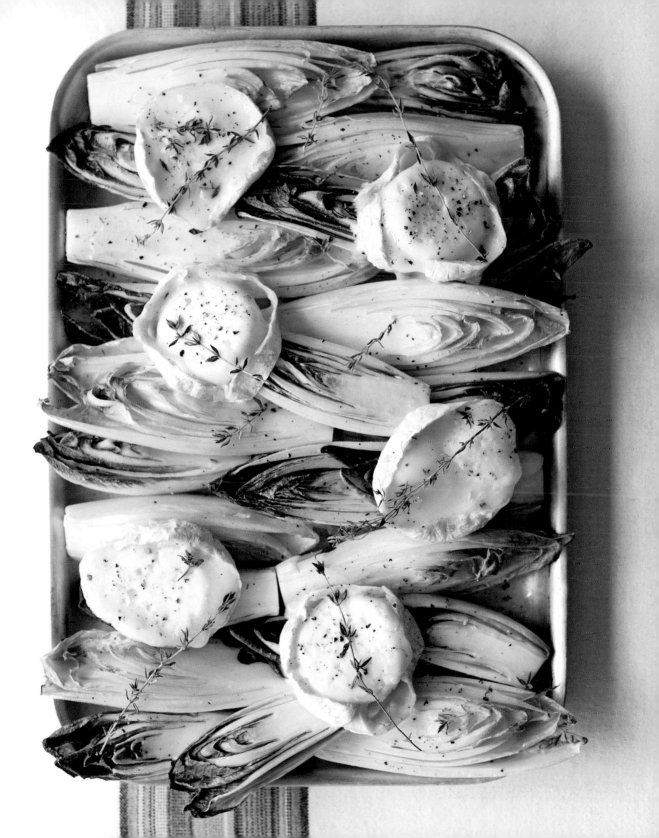

Orecchiette alla Pugliese

Another great, healthy pasta dish, this time from Puglia in southern Italy. Traditionally, the Italians make this with a kind of broccoli called *rapini*. It's hard to find in Britain, but our sprouting broccoli makes a great substitute.

serves 2
prep time 5 minutes
cooking time 15 minutes
255 calories per serving

200g sprouting broccoli, trimmed and chopped into 2cm pieces
125g orecchiette pasta
extra-virgin olive oil spray
2 cloves of garlic, peeled and finely chopped
1 mild red chilli, deseeded and finely chopped
salt and pepper

Boil the broccoli in salted water for about 3 minutes until it's just yielding. Drain, refresh in cold water and set aside to dry.
Cook the orecchiette according to the packet instructions until al dente. Heat a spritz of olive oil in a non-stick frying pan. Add the garlic and the chilli. When the garlic is just starting to colour, add the broccoli. Sauté for about 5 minutes until cooked. Season with salt and pepper.
Add the broccoli to the cooked and drained orecchiette. Spritz once again with olive oil, stir together and serve.

tip

For extra savoury depth, add two or three drained, chopped anchovy fillets to the oil when sautéing the garlic and chilli.

Oven-roasted ratatouille with brown rice

This is a really easy and fresh version of the traditional classic, which removes an awful lot of the hard work – and a lot of the fat!

serves 2
prep time 10–15 minutes
cooking time 30–40 minutes
302 calories per serving

1 courgette, sliced
4 vine tomatoes, halved
1 small aubergine, cubed
1 red onion, cut into 8 chunks
1 yellow pepper, deseeded and cut into chunks
2 cloves of garlic, peeled and sliced
extra-virgin olive oil spray
1 teaspoon herbes de Provence
salt and pepper
50ml white wine
100g brown rice
150ml chicken stock (home-made if possible)
a handful of fresh basil, shredded

Preheat the oven to 200°C/fan 180°C.
Place the courgette, tomatoes, aubergine, onion, yellow pepper and garlic in a roasting tin. Spritz with the olive oil spray. Sprinkle over the herbes de Provence and season with salt and pepper. Mix well, and pour over the wine.
Put in the oven for about 30 to 40 minutes.
Meanwhile, put the brown rice and stock into a large pan, add a pinch of salt and bring to the boil. Once the water is boiling, turn the heat right down and put the lid on the rice. Leave to simmer for 20 to 25 minutes. Turn the heat off, drain the rice and let it sit until the vegetable are ready. Remove the vegetables from the oven, adjust the seasoning and stir in the fresh basil.
Serve piping hot with the rice.

This is also great cold with salad, as a sandwich or as a topping for baked potatoes.

Fusilli con zucchini e pomodori

This is a delicious and simple courgette and tomato pasta dish from Campagna in southern Italy. It's an area often associated with seafood, but it is also famous for its vegetables and salads. This sauce really brings out the rich, sunny flavour of both the cherry tomatoes and the courgettes.

serves 4
prep time 10 minutes
cooking time 25 minutes
197 calories per serving

1 small onion, chopped
extra-virgin olive oil spray
1 clove garlic, peeled and crushed
1 × 400g can chopped tomatoes
1 tablespoon tomato purée
1 teaspoon dried basil
1 teaspoon dried oregano
a dash of white wine
salt and pepper
125g fusilli pasta
2 small courgettes, topped and tailed and sliced
16 cherry tomatoes
a handful of fresh basil leaves
4 tablespoons grated Parmesan cheese

You can use any shape of pasta you like. Be sure to check the individual packets for cooking times, as they will all be different. There is no need to add oil to the pasta water. It will only rise to the surface and is a waste of precious calories!

Sauté the onion in a spray of olive oil until it starts to soften and colour. Add the garlic and cook for a further 2 minutes. Add the can of tomatoes, the tomato purée, the dried herbs and the wine, and season with salt and pepper.
Stir the sauce well and allow it to simmer for 10 minutes.
While the sauce is cooking, add the fusilli to a large pan of boiling salted water and cook according to the instructions on the packet or until al dente.
Add the courgettes and cherry tomatoes to the sauce and cook until they are just soft – another 4 minutes.
Shred the basil leaves, stir through the sauce, and serve over the drained fusilli with up to a tablespoon of Parmesan cheese.

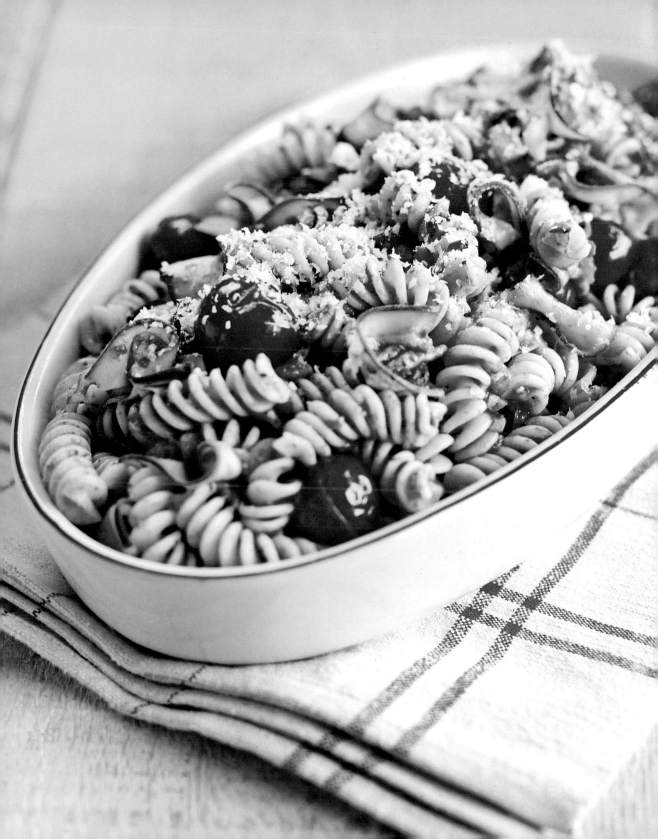

Stuffed butternut squash with sweet peppers

Here's a yummy squash stuffed with peas and beans, and flavoured with saffron.

serves 4
prep time: 20 minutes
cooking time 1–1½ hours
163 calories per serving

1 butternut squash, halved and deseeded
extra-virgin olive oil spray
1 onion, finely chopped
1 × 410g can of cannellini beans, drained and rinsed
1 red pepper, deseeded and diced
½ yellow pepper, deseeded and diced
1 clove of garlic, peeled and finely chopped

80g peas, fresh or frozen
a pinch of saffron, soaked in 2 teaspoons of hot water
a pinch of grated nutmeg
a few drops of balsamic vinegar
salt and pepper
1 tablespoon fresh parsley, chopped
1 tablespoon grated Parmesan
½ slice Swedish-style rye bread, whizzed into crumbs

Preheat the oven to 170°C/fan 150°C.
Place the halved squash, cut sides uppermost, on a baking tray. Spray your palm once with olive oil for each half, and rub into the squash. Precook the squash in the oven for 30–50 minutes, until barely tender.
Heat a spray of oil in a saucepan and soften the onion.
Drain and rinse the beans. Pulse briefly in a food processor or just mash with a fork – break them up a bit, don't reduce to a paste. Set aside.
Add the peppers, the garlic and the peas to the onion. Add the saffron and its liquid, the nutmeg and the balsamic vinegar, and cook gently for 7 minutes. Season with salt and plenty of black pepper, and add the parsley. Stir the cooked vegetables into the cannellini beans and set aside.
Mix the Parmesan, breadcrumbs and a spray of oil in a bowl.
When the squash is tender, remove it from the oven. Spoon out the flesh above the seed hole, leaving about a 1cm thickness of the sweet, golden flesh remaining against the skin.
Chop the squash you have removed as finely as you can, and stir it into the vegetable mixture.
Now fill each half of the squash with the stuffing mixture. Sprinkle over the Parmesan and rye breadcrumb topping, and bake in the oven for a further 20 to 30 minutes or until golden brown. Serve piping hot.

tip

We love spaghetti squash too, because of its crazy string-like interior. You could also use acorn squash, turban squash – any of them, in fact. You will be amazed if you visit a local farmers' market, especially in the autumn, at all the different and beautiful shapes, colours and varieties of squash.

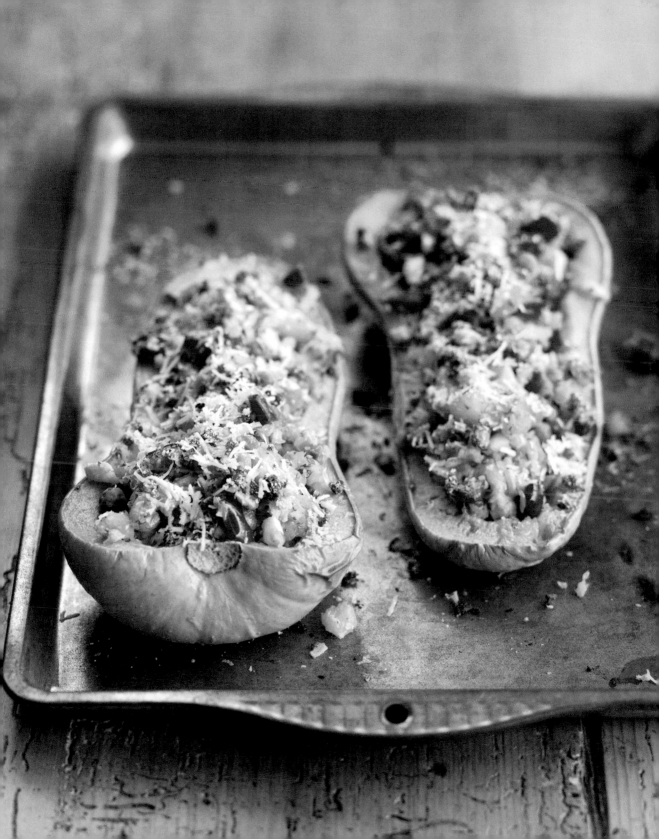

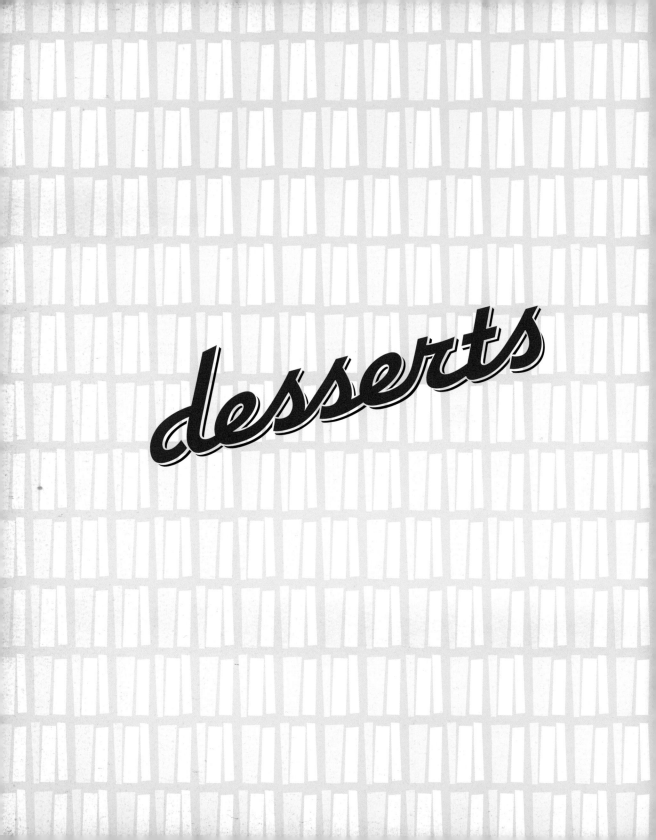

desserts

If you thought Cooking Yourself Thin was going to mean a life without desserts, then think again! Often loaded with fat and sugar, these are the foods we love to eat, but hate to love. The good news is that by using these recipes, which are all calorie controlled, you can still include delicious puddings into your plan without feeling guilty. We've allowed up to 200 calories a day for treats or dessert, so if you have a sweet tooth, remember to leave room for treats when planning your meals.

Banana loaf

Tasty, moist and low in fat, this cake is a favourite with everyone.

makes 14 slices
prep time 20 minutes
cooking time 1 hour 15 minutes
201 calories per slice

50g butter
175g light brown soft sugar
2 medium free-range eggs, lightly beaten
350g peeled ripe bananas, mashed
200g self-raising flour sifted
½ teaspoon salt
½ teaspoon bicarbonate of soda
75g walnuts, roughly chopped
6 walnut halves

Preheat the oven to 180°C/fan 160°C. Line and grease a 1kg loaf tin.
Cream the butter with the sugar in a large mixing bowl until the mixture is light and fluffy.
Add the beaten eggs, and gradually whisk them into the butter and sugar.
Add the mashed bananas and beat the mixture well.
Carefully fold in the flour, salt and bicarbonate of soda. Stir in the walnuts.
Put the cake mixture into the prepared loaf tin and decorate with the walnut halves, pressing them gently into the mixture.
Bake for 1 hour to 1 hour 15 minutes, until the cake has risen and is golden. Allow to cool.
Like all freshly baked loaves, this banana loaf looks best served on a breadboard with a knife for people to help themselves. This recipe is good eaten the next day too.

tip
To reduce the calories even more, you can use a sugar substitute. To mash the bananas, we always use our hands!

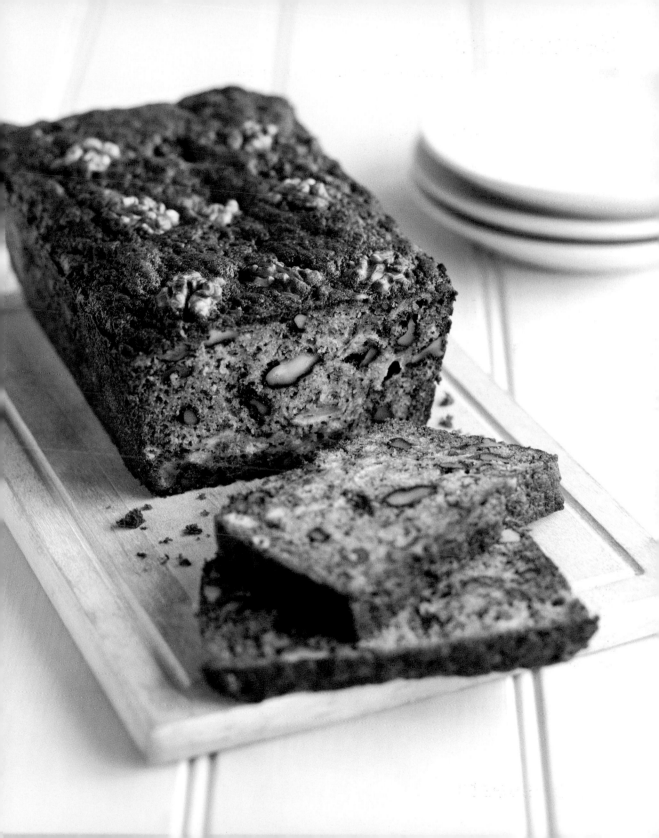

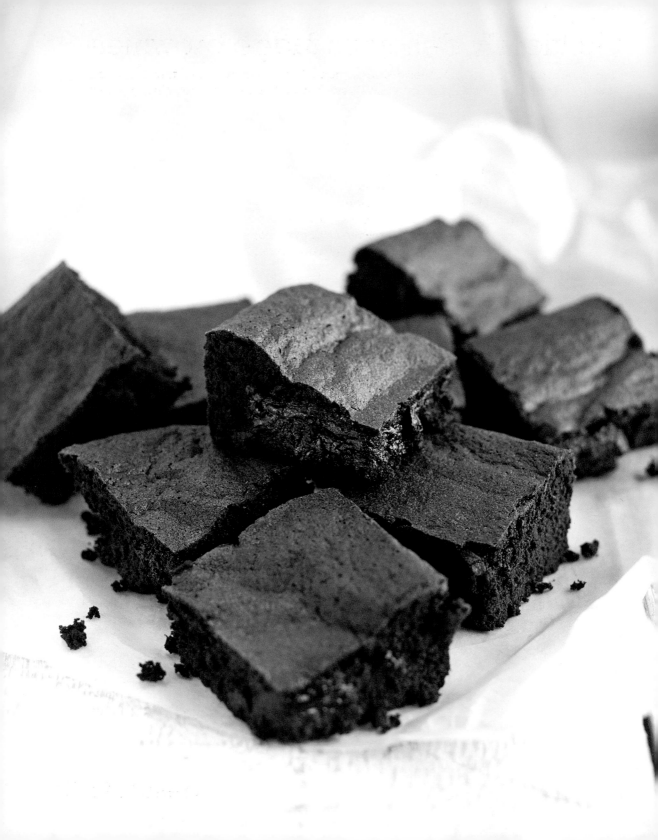

Guiltlessly delicious fudge brownies

These squashy, chocolaty brownies are so gorgeously rich, you will think they are loaded with fat and calories. But they're not! They're lower in fat than regular brownies, and they're lower in sugar too!

makes 18–20 brownies
prep time 10 minutes
cooking time 15 minutes
82 calories per brownie (20 brownies)
86 calories per brownie (19 brownies)
91 calories per brownie (18 brownies)

50ml vegetable, sunflower or safflower oil
150g white caster sugar
2 medium free-range eggs, well beaten
1 teaspoon vanilla extract
50g cocoa powder
½ teaspoon baking powder
80g plain flour

Preheat the oven to 175°C/fan 155°C.
In a large bowl, mix together the oil and sugar. Add the eggs and vanilla and stir vigorously until well blended.
Carefully add the cocoa powder with the baking powder and flour, and mix well.
Grease and flour a 20 × 20cm baking pan and pour the batter into the tin, using a spatula to make sure you clean the bowl.
Bake for approximately 15 minutes or until done. A cocktail stick inserted in the centre should come out with a few very slightly moist crumbs on it. That means your brownies are done, but will still have that gooey, fudgy texture.
Chocolate brownies are yummy hot or cold, and can be served just as they are or with some low-fat vanilla ice cream for a special treat.

tip
Putting the brownies in the fridge will keep them fresh for up to a week… if they last that long! They also freeze well.

Amaretto-amaretti peaches

This Italian dessert is easy to make, weighs in really low in fat, and looks as spectacular as it tastes. It can be made in advance and kept cold in the fridge. This is a winner whenever we serve it. Bellissimo!

serves 6
prep time 20 minutes
cooking time 35–40 minutes
180 calories per serving

6 ripe peaches
6 amaretti biscuits
200ml Marsala wine
100ml Amaretto liqueur
3 tablespoons caster sugar
½ cinnamon stick or ½ teaspoon ground cinnamon
1 vanilla pod, halved lengthways
star anise (optional)

Preheat the oven to 170°C/fan 150°C.
Cut the peaches in half, remove the stones and lay, cut side up, in a shallow ovenproof dish.
Crumble the amaretti biscuits into the hollows left by the stones.
Pour the Marsala, Amaretto and sugar into a small saucepan and heat gently, stirring, until the sugar has dissolved. Add the cinnamon, vanilla and star anise (if using) to the liquid, and leave to infuse for as long as possible.
Pour the liquid over the peaches and bake for 45 minutes. Check the peaches halfway through cooking and baste with the liquid.
Leave to cool and put in the fridge to chill until needed.
Place in serving bowls with some of the boozy juices spooned over.

tip

You could easily use another fruit: peaches, plums, figs and bananas are all delicious when baked. And try experimenting with different liqueurs: Tia Maria, rum, Grand Marnier or Frangelico.

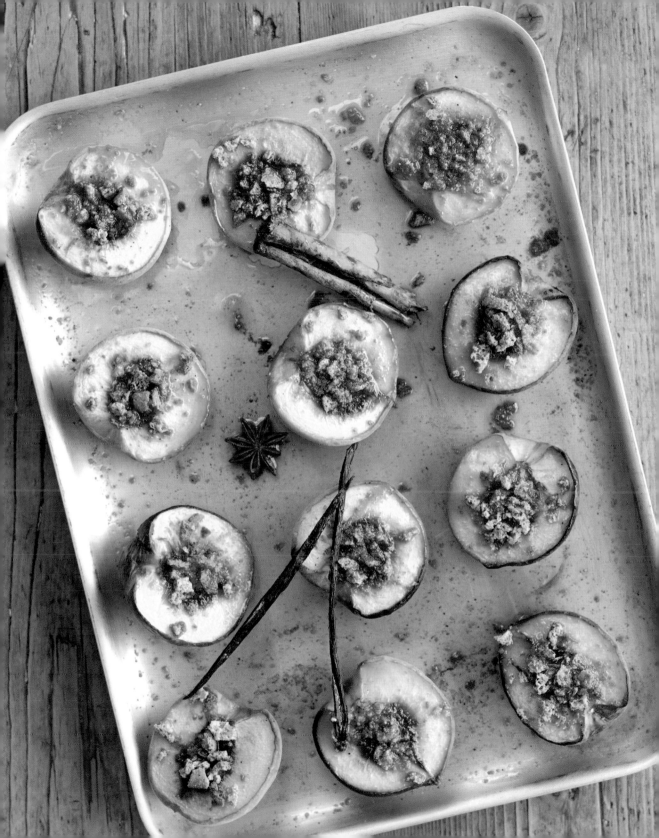

Raspberry jelly trifle

It's the ultimate quick and easy recipe – this won't take you any time at all to throw together. This yummy summery dessert is easy to make, looks fabulous, and won't leave you feeling stuffed to the gills!

serves 4
prep time 3–4 minutes plus 3 hours setting time
37 calories per serving

23g packet sugar-free raspberry jelly
250g punnet of raspberries
40g light aerosol cream

Make up the raspberry jelly as per the packet instructions.
Put a handful of raspberries in each of four glasses and pour over the prepared jelly in equal portions.
Place in the fridge to set.
Once set, pipe over small swirls of aerosol cream.
We like to serve this in large wine glasses. Enjoy!

tip

Why not spice things up by mixing the jelly with a spirit of your choice? If you use spirits, put the jelly in the freezer to set.

Couscous cake

This recipe is super-easy – it's a case of throwing everything into one bowl and baking the results. The end result is a great-tasting cake that will remind you of bread pudding. We love sitting around chatting with friends, with a huge cup of tea and a big wedge of this cake.

serves 6
prep time 10 minutes
cooking time 40 minutes
181 calories per serving (25g sultanas)
192 calories per serving (50g sultanas)

200g couscous
oil spray
2 × 200g low-fat yoghurts (under 100 calories and any flavour
  – our favourite is a combination of 1 plain and 1 toffee)
1 teaspoon mixed spice
25–50g sultanas
10g granulated sweetener

Preheat the oven to 200°C/fan 180°C.
Make up the couscous according to the packet instructions, and spritz lightly with oil.
Add all the other ingredients to the couscous and mix well.
Spoon the mixture into a 20 × 20cm cake tin, flattening the top with a spatula. Bake in the oven for 40 minutes until golden brown. Serve immediately as a nice warm treat with a scoop of low-fat ice cream, or leave to cool and chill in the fridge.

Make sure the sweetener you use is one that's safe to bake with, like Splenda. To make a Bakewell tart version, try cherry yoghurts, replace the sultanas with glace cherries and add a teaspoon of vanilla essence.

Marshmallow fruit salad with frozen vanilla yoghurt

This sweet snack will squelch your sugar cravings in just a few minutes. We prepare a few portions of frozen yoghurt beforehand so it's in the freezer for when we need it.

serves 2
prep time 10 minutes plus 3 hours freezing time
100 calories per serving

100g low-fat live, natural yoghurt
1 teaspoon vanilla extract
2 teaspoons honey
5 sugar-free marshmallows
100g strawberries
50g blueberries
50g raspberries

Mix the yoghurt, vanilla extract and honey thoroughly with a spoon in a plastic pot.
Freeze the yoghurt mixture for at least 3 hours in your freezer, beating halfway through the freezing time to break down the ice crystals.
Snip the marshmallows into small pieces with dampened scissors, and put the bits in a dessert bowl.
Rinse the fruit gently. Remove the hulls from the strawberries and cut them into four pieces. Mix all the fruit with the marshmallows.
Arrange scoops of the frozen yoghurt on top of the fruit salad.

This is lovely with a cup of mint tea garnished with a slice of lemon.

Chocolate crispy cakes

OK, so these aren't exactly healthy, but at less than 100 calories a cake, they're wonderful for a luxurious treat once in a while, and will keep in the fridge for ages.

 makes 20–26 cakes
prep time 10 minutes
65–84 calories per cake, dependent on quantities made

200g good-quality milk chocolate
1 tablespoon clear honey
150g Rice Krispies

Break the chocolate into small pieces and melt in a bowl over a saucepan of boiling water. Stir to help the chocolate melt.
When the chocolate is almost fully melted, stir in the honey and take it off the heat (the chocolate will continue to melt because the bowl is hot, you don't want to burn it).
Stir in the Rice Krispies, a handful at a time, and ensure they are fully coated in the chocolate mixture.
Spoon the mixture into cake cases. These amounts should make between twenty and twenty-six if you don't overfill the cases. Leave to set in the fridge for an hour or so.

Eton mess

This creamy, crunchy dessert is totally sublime and can be made in under 5 minutes. You need to eat up, though, because Eton mess doesn't keep for more than a few hours once assembled.

serves 4
prep time 5 minutes
170 calories per serving

6 × 16g meringue nests
100g vanilla yoghurt
50g half-fat crème fraîche
1 teaspoon vanilla extract
400g hulled strawberries
3 sprigs of mint

Take a large bowl and crumble the meringue nests into it, making sure some of the pieces are at least 1cm square.
Stir in the yoghurt, crème fraîche and vanilla extract.
Crush about half of the strawberries with a fork and cut the remainder into bite-sized pieces. Stir these into the meringue mix.
Serve in pretty individual bowls with a sprig of fresh mint.

tip

If you can be patient, then leave the dessert for about 1 hour before eating it. The smaller pieces of meringue start softening and you get a gorgeous gradation of crunchiness to complement the creaminess.

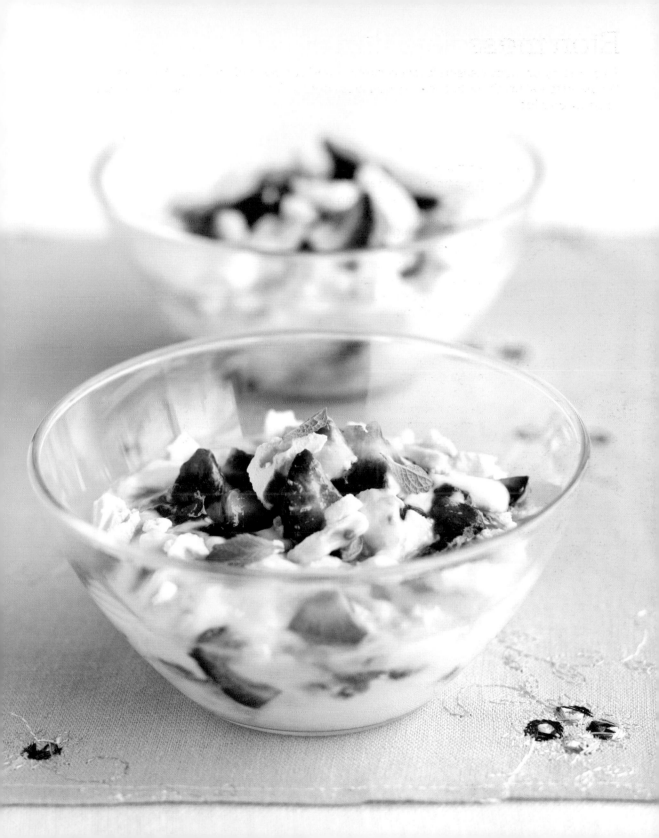

Dark chocolate and coffee mousse

Everyone loves a chocolate hit at the end of a meal, and this light mousse delivers in spades. It's also about as healthy as a chocolate pud can be – no butter, no cream, just a solid chocolate whack to the taste buds! Make sure you buy the best chocolate and the best eggs you can find.

serves 4
prep time 10 minutes plus 3 hours chilling
cooking time 4–5 minutes
139 calories per serving

75g good-quality plain chocolate (at least 70% cocoa solids)
1 shot of espresso
2 medium eggs
1 teaspoon caster sugar

Melt the chocolate in a bowl over boiling water. Stir the espresso into the melted chocolate (you can use decaf if you like) and remove from the heat.
Separate the eggs. Whisk the whites into stiff peaks in a clean bowl, then fold in the sugar.
Beat the egg yolks and mix them into the chocolate.
Fold the egg whites into this mixture very gently.
Place the mixture carefully into individual ramekins or espresso cups.
Chill in the fridge for about 3 hours or overnight until set.

Try leaving out the espresso and adding the grated zest of an orange and a splash of orange juice. Don't serve dishes containing raw eggs to pregnant or breast-feeding women, small children or the elderly.

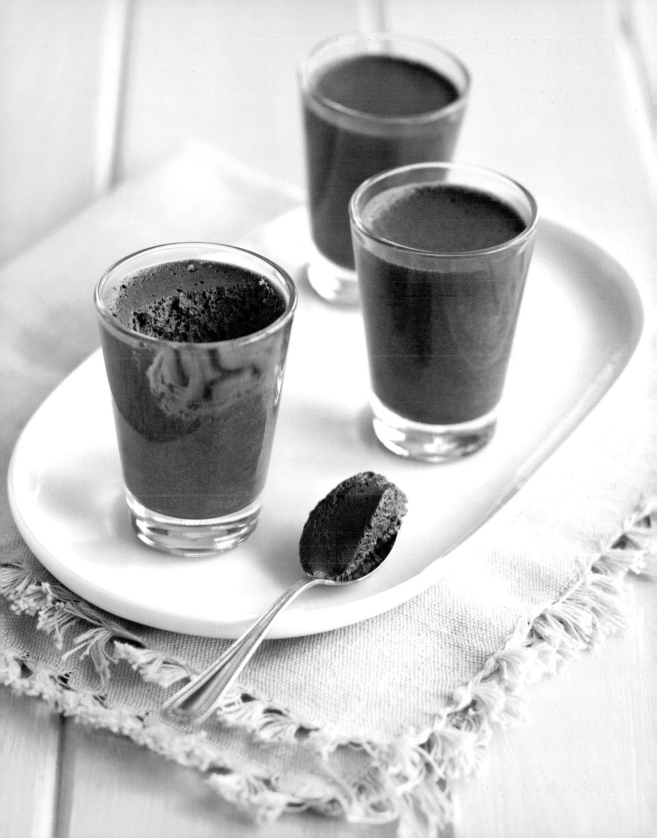

Light strawberry sponge

This is a light and easy sponge cake recipe. The filling can be adapted to whatever you fancy, and so can look quite impressive. This serves ten, but the recipe can easily be halved if you don't think your willpower can cope with having the whole cake in the house! It is great for summer parties or even afternoon tea.

serves 10
prep time 20 minutes
cooking time 20 minutes
187 calories per serving

4 large free-range eggs, separated
160g light granulated sugar
1 teaspoon vanilla extract
110g plain flour
100ml whipping cream
200g strawberries, hulled and sliced
icing sugar

Preheat the oven to 190°C/fan 170°C.
Line the base of two 20cm round sandwich tins, then grease and lightly flour the sides and base.
Beat the egg yolks with the sugar in a mixing bowl for 6 to 8 minutes (do this gently to begin with), then add 4 tablespoons of warm water. Continue to beat for another 8 minutes until the mixture is very pale and fluffy and leaves the trail of the whisk for at least 10 seconds. Fold in the vanilla extract.
Sift the flour onto a plate. Lightly fold the flour into the egg yolk mixture, a few spoonfuls at a time.
In a separate bowl, whisk the egg whites until soft peaks form and then fold the egg whites through the mixture. Remember to do this gently.
Pour the mixture out into the tin and bake for 20 minutes or until the sponge springs back when gently pushed and is golden brown.
Turn out onto racks to cool. When completely cool, whip the cream to a smooth, thick consistency.
Halve the strawberries. Spread half the cream on the bottom layer of the cake and arrange the strawberries on this layer. Top with the remaining cream.
Place the top layer of the cake on top of the filling, and dust the top with icing sugar.

tip

Use an electric whisk for the cream and egg whites. You can also use one for the yolks and sugar, but mix with a fork first. If you have any leftover strawberries, serve them on the side and enjoy!

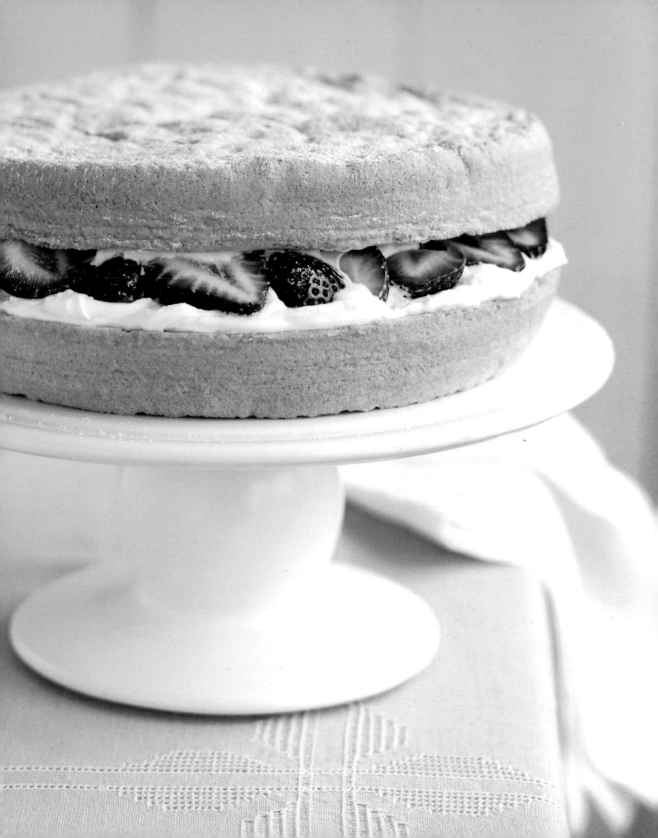

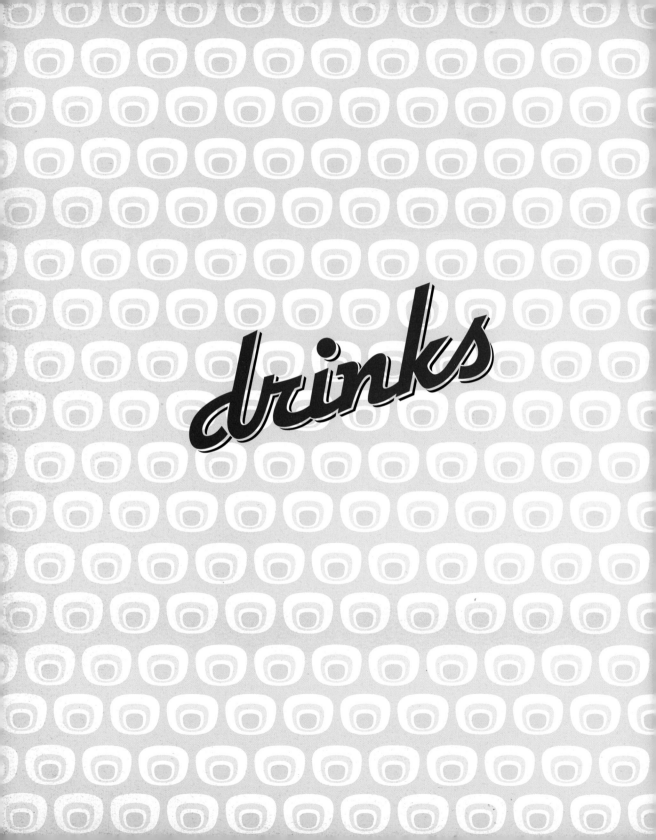

drinks

These recipes for cool cocktails should be up everyone's sleeve. Alcohol is second only to fat in the amount of calories it provides, so quality rather than quantity is the answer here. Soft drinks and trendy coffees are two other big offenders, so our healthier suggestions are an easy way to ditch some empty calories.

Peach mojito

A fresh, sweet summer drink, perfect at a barbecue, or for just relaxing in the garden by yourself

serves 2
prep time 3–5 minutes
60 calories per glass

1 large sprig of mint
1 teaspoon caster sugar or sweetener
¼ lime
crushed ice
25ml white rum
25ml peach schnapps
400ml soda water

Combine the mint leaves, sugar and lime in a cocktail shaker. Use the end of a rolling pin to muddle (bash and mix) them together.
Add a handful of crushed ice, the rum and schnapps. Place the lid on the shaker and give it all a good shake.
Divide the mix between two glasses and top up with soda water.
Serve with a straw!

Zinc bar punch

This tropical cocktail hails (strangely) from France. The islands of the French Caribbean, most notably Martinique and Guadeloupe, make some terrific rum, perfect for cocktails. One zinc bar we know down on the coast of Provence steeps juices for its punch in a massive bar-top bell jar. This is as close as we've come to recreating it. It's delicious, and a just a little bit lethal!

serves 2
prep time 15 minutes (longer if you have the time as it just gets better!)
132 calories per glass

50ml freshly squeezed orange juice
50ml unsweetened mango juice
50ml unsweetened guava juice
a generous grating of nutmeg
4 crushed allspice berries
4 whole cloves
crushed ice
100ml white rum, preferably from Martinique or Guadeloupe
1 lime, cut into quarters

Mix the fruit juices together in a jug and add the spices. Leave to stand for as long as you can – it will keep for up to a week in the fridge and be all the better for it. Alternatively, and because time is often short, you can get away with 15 to 20 minutes.
Fill two glasses with the ice. Pour 50ml of rum into each glass. Cut the lime into quarters. Top up with the fruit juices, pouring through a tea strainer to keep out the cloves and shards of allspice.
Squeeze a quarter of lime into each of the glasses and enjoy the cocktail while it's cold!

Bellini cardinale

This is a delicious summer cocktail. The purée takes a little effort, but it's worth it for such a pretty and refreshing drink.

serves 6
prep time 10 minutes
107 calories per glass

50g strawberries, hulled
200g raspberries
a squeeze of lemon
1 teaspoon icing sugar
1 × 75cl bottle of Prosecco

Use the back of a spoon to push the strawberries and raspberries through a fine sieve, turning them into a purée. This is very important, if a bit laborious, because pips just ruin the fun.
Add the lemon juice and sugar to the purée and stir well.
To serve, pour a good dash of the purée into the bottom of a chilled champagne flute. Top up with chilled Prosecco (be careful – it will fizz up like crazy).
The ideal proportions of purée to Prosecco are 1:5.

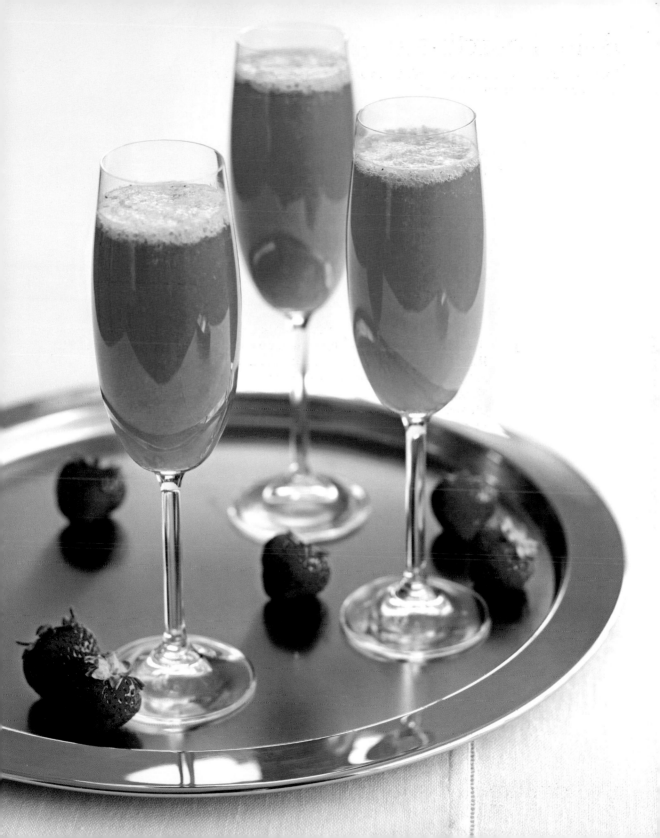

Home-made limeade

Refreshingly simple, and simply refreshing!

serves 1
prep time 5 minutes
9 calories per glass using sugar
2 calories per glass using sweetener

juice of 1 lime
½ teaspoon sugar or sweetener
ice
fizzy water

Pour the lime juice into a tall glass with 1 tablespoon of hot water
and the sugar. Stir until all the sugar dissolves.
Fill the glass with ice and then top up with fizzy water.

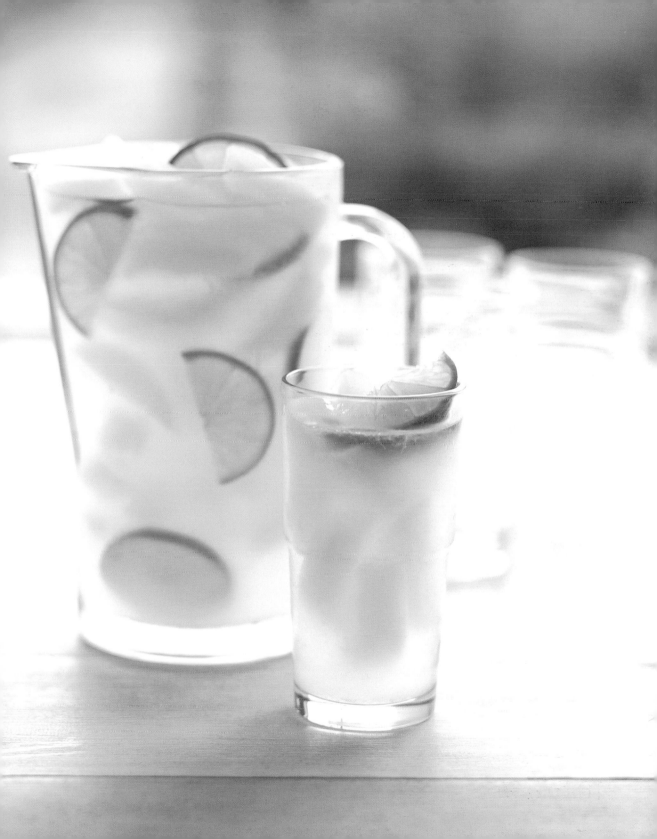

Iced cardamom coffee

Cardamom goes beautifully with coffee. It's a famous combination throughout the Middle East; the spicy perfume of the cardamom marrying elegantly with the bitterness of the coffee. Arabic coffee is often served ferociously sweet. This iced coffee includes just the tiniest bit of sugar to take the edge off.

serves 1
prep time 3 minutes
57 calories per glass

1 teaspoon cardamom pods
ground coffee (enough for one 50–60ml espresso shot)
ice
125ml skimmed milk
1 teaspoon sugar to taste

Swap the sugar for sweetener and save 16 calories per glass.

Crush the cardamom pods with the back of a knife to release the seeds. Mix the cardamom with the coffee grounds and make a shot of espresso. Fill a glass with ice.
Pour in half the milk, then strain the coffee and add along with the rest of the milk. Stir well. Add the sugar, stir again, and enjoy.

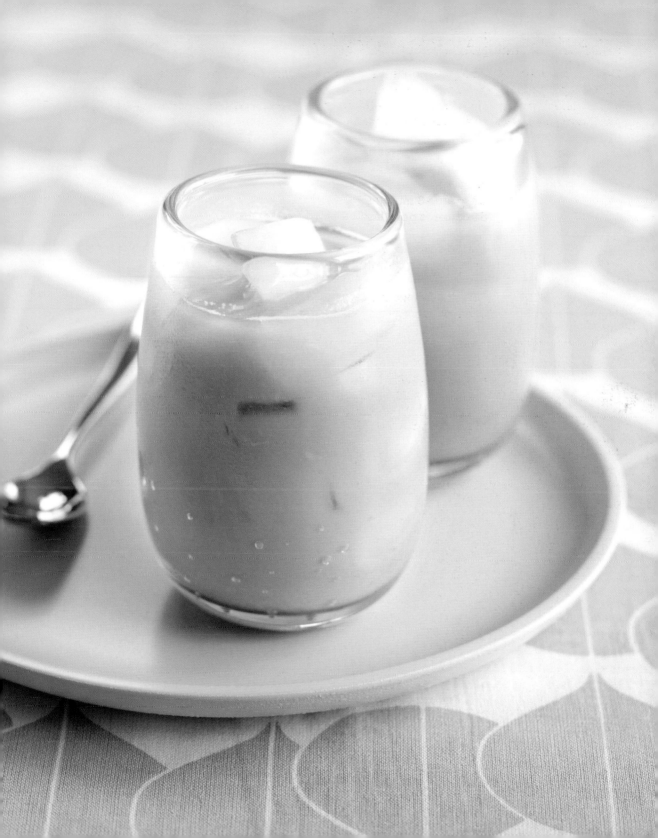

The Homewood

A deliciously fresh, low-alcohol cooler for a hot summer's day.

serves 1
prep time 2–3 minutes
66 calories per glass

100ml fizzy water
crushed ice
a dash of Angostura bitters
200ml grapefruit juice (preferably freshly squeezed)

Angostura bitters are another great store-cupboard staple. A few splashes will give depth of flavour to shepherd's pie, beef stews and soups, as well as adding a sophisticated twist to cold drinks and cocktails.

Pour the fizzy water into a glass over ice. Add a good dash of Angostura bitters, and then top up with the grapefruit juice.

Dips and dressings

If the salad leaves, crudités or toasted pitta soldiers are the body, then dressings and dips are the clothing! You can be as casual as you want, or exotic and glamorous! All of these recipes dress one large salad or make dips for one or two people.

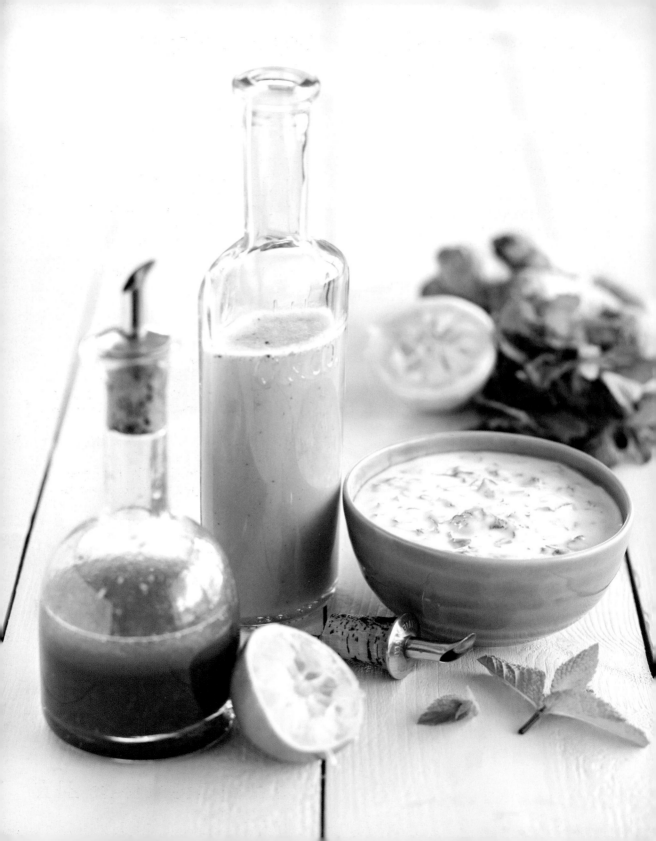

Yogurt raita dressing

Creamy and smooth, this salad is great for cooling down a curry.

48 calories
2 tablespoons low-fat yogurt
a handful of fresh mint, torn
1 tablespoon lemon juice
a good pinch of salt

Combine all the ingredients and use to dress leafy salads or cooked lentils. Serve alongside grilled meats or curry.

Honey and mustard dressing

This is great with a ham or gammon salad. Beautifully British!

132 calories
1 teaspoon cider vinegar
salt and freshly ground black pepper
a pinch of ground mace
1 teaspoon vegetable oil
1 tablespoon English mustard
1 tablespoon runny honey

Mix the vinegar, salt, pepper and mace together. Add the oil. Add the mustard and the honey and combine well.

Soy and ginger dressing

This is great with steamed Asian vegetables, salmon salad or a pea shoot and asparagus salad.

34 calories
1 tablespoon light soy sauce
2 teaspoons lime juice
½ teaspoon finely grated fresh ginger
1 teaspoon vegetable oil
freshly ground black pepper

Whisk all the ingredients together, and you're ready to go!

Salsa cruda

Instead of dipping greasy tortilla chips, try crisp baked pitta bread with this sunny salsa.

65 calories
4 tomatoes, roughly chopped
1 serrano chilli, deseeded (the big green or red ones you get in the supermarket are fine)
a handful of fresh coriander, chopped
juice of ½ lime
a pinch of sea salt

Mix all the ingredients together in a pretty bowl and serve immediately.

Smoky chipotle dip

Chipotle chillies are a smoked, dried Mexican variety, and they're simply stunning. You can buy them in the UK from The Cool Chile Company or **www.mexgrocer.co.uk**, bottled or canned in a rich tomato sauce called *adobo*. And they're well worth looking for: they last for ages in the fridge and add an incredible depth of smoky, spicy heat to lots of dishes!

100 calories
1 tinned chipotle chilli in *adobo* sauce
1 teaspoon *adobo* sauce
4 tablespoons low-fat soured cream
   or 0% fat Greek yoghurt
a pinch of salt

Chop the chilli finely. Mix in the teaspoon of *adobo* sauce and the soured cream. Add a little salt and serve with crudités (endives and sweet peppers are good) and pitta chips.

If you're worried that the dip will be too spicy, start by stirring the *adobo* sauce into the soured cream or yoghurt without the chopped chilli. Add the chilli bit by bit, tasting as you go.

Healthy houmous

We know you worry about the fat in houmous, so here is our lower-fat version. This makes a fair bit, but it keeps well in the fridge, and is great on spuds or in sandwiches.

313 calories
1 × 410g tin chickpeas, drained and rinsed
juice of ½ lemon
1 clove of garlic
sea salt
½ teaspoon ground cumin
½ teaspoon cayenne pepper
1 teaspoon extra-virgin olive oil

Put everything in the blender with 3 tablespoons of water and whiz until smooth. Add a little more water or lemon juice if it seems too thick.
Serve with a light dusting of cayenne pepper and another drizzle of olive oil.

Index

Amaretto-amaretti peaches 192, **193**
apples
    roast beetroot and apple soup 82, 83
    sweet potato and apple soup 79
    warm chicken liver and apple
        salad 107
artichokes
    Jerusalem artichoke soup 85
asparagus
    garden-fresh quiche 162, **163**
    roast asparagus on rocket with a
        Parmesan vinaigrette 176, **177**
avocados
    marmite and avocado on toast 78
    prawn, avocado and mango wraps
        with coriander 60

bacon
    broad bean and bacon risotto 113
    roast bacon, tomatoes and mushrooms
        with parsley gremolata 42, **43**
baked goat's cheese and chicory salad
    178, **179**
baked potatoes *see* jacket potatoes
banana(s)
    chocolate-banana sunflower muffins
        69, **68**
    coconut and banana pancakes 38, **39**
    kiwi, banana and lime sunshine
        smoothie 36
    loaf 188, **189**
    Mo'Bay smoothie 37
beans
    broad bean and bacon risotto 113
    cod saltimbocca 146, **147**
    harissa-spiced chicken with bean
        and couscous salad 100, **101**
    stuffed butternut squash with sweet
        peppers 184, **185**
    Texas chilli con carne 131
beef
    beer marinade for steak 118
    Louisiana-style zesty burgers 135, **134**
    rare beef with horseradish and
        watercress on wholemeal 54
    shin and mushroom casserole 127
    Texas chilli con carne 131
    Vietnamese beef and mint salad 57, **56**
beer marinade for steak 118
beetroot
    beetroot, mint and feta topping for
        jacket potato 170
    roast beetroot and apple soup 82, **83**
Bellini cardinale 208, **209**
braised lamb shanks 132, **133**
bread
    poached egg with smoked trout
        on wholemeal toast 44
    see also sandwiches; toast; wraps

broad bean and bacon risotto 113
broccoli
    garden-fresh quiche 162, **163**
    orecchiette alla Pugliese 180
brownies 191, **190**
burgers
    Louisiana-style zesty 135, **134**
butternut squash *see* squash

cakes
    banana loaf 188, **189**
    chocolate crispy 197
    couscous 195
    fudge brownies 191, **190**
    strawberry sponge 202, **203**
    see also muffins
calories 9
capers 122
    piquant marinade for fish 118
    tuna, spring onions, lemon, pepper
        and capers toping for jacket
        potatoes 170
cardamom
    iced cardamom coffee 212, **213**
    -scented basmati rice 173
carrots
    spiced carrot and orange soup 84
cashew nuts
    chickpea, spinach and cashew nut
        korma with pilaf 166, **167**
casserole
    beef shin and mushroom 127
cauliflower and pasta cheese bake 165
celeriac soup 85
cheese
    baked goat's cheese and chicory
        salad 178, **179**
    beetroot, mint and feta topping for
        jacket potato 170
    cauliflower and pasta cheese bake 165
    club wrap 60
    Greek salad 62, **63**
    halloumi and tomato kebabs 130
    roast asparagus on rocket with a
        Parmesan vinaigrette 176, **177**
    tricolore topping for jacket potato 170
chicken
    Catalan 90—1, **91**
    Coronation chicken salad 67
    creamy chicken curry 94
    creamy lemon-coriander chicken
        curry with red peppers 96, **97**
    five-spice chicken with a vegetable
        stir-fry 93, **92**
    harissa-spiced chicken with bean
        and couscous salad 100, **101**
    jerked chicken with fresh mango
        salsa 106
    maple syrup 99, **98**

    and mushroom curry 103
    and mushroom risotto 104, **105**
    Southern wild rice and Cajun
        chicken salad 61
    spicy marinade for 118
    tarragon 95
chicken livers
    warm chicken liver and apple salad 107
chickpeas
    chickpea, spinach and cashew nut
        korma with pilaf 166, **167**
    homous 218
chicory
    baked goat's cheese and chicory
        salad 178, **179**
chilli con carne, Texas 131
chillies
    hot-and-sour prawn noodle 86, **87**
    salsa cruda 217
    smoky chipotle dip 218
    spicy Thai butternut squash soup 75
chipotle dip, smoky 218
chives
    pastry-free chive and onion quiche 172
chocolate
    -banana sunflower muffins 69, **68**
    crispy cakes 197
    dark chocolate and coffee mousse
        200, **201**
coconut and banana pancakes 38, **39**
cod
    saltimbocca 146, **147**
    seafood lasagne 140, **141**
coffee
    dark chocolate and coffee mousse
        200, **201**
    iced cardamom 212, **213**
coleslaw 126
coley, spicy Italian 142, **143**
compote
    red berry compote with yoghurt
        and honey 40
coriander
    creamy lemon-coriander chicken
        curry with red peppers 96, **97**
    prawn, avocado and mango wraps
        with 60
    Puy lentil and coriander salad 65
    salsa cruda 217
corned beef
    panackelty 112
coronation chicken salad 67
courgettes
    fusilli con zucchini e pomodori 182, **183**
couscous
    harissa-spiced chicken with bean
        and couscous salad 100, **101**
    prawn and parsley couscous salad 55
couscous cake 195

Page numbers in **bold** denote an illustration

crayfish
    lemony-garlic crayfish and pea
        shoots on rye 54
cream cheese
    wrap-around Manhattan 60
crème frâiche
    Eton mess 198, **199**
    Normandy pork fillet 136, **137**
    tarragon chicken 95
cucumbers
    Greek salad 62, **63**
    sardines with cucumber, lemon
        and flat-leaf parsley on toast 78
cumin
    Maltese pea and cumin soup 80
curry
    chicken and mushroom 103
    chickpea, spinach and cashew nut
        korma with pilaf 166, **167**
    creamy chicken 94
    creamy lemon-coriander chicken
        curry with red peppers 96, **97**

dahl with okra and sweet potato 173
desserts
    Amaretto-amaretti peaches 192, **193**
    dark chocolate and coffee mousse
        200, **201**
    Eton mess 198, **199**
    marshmallow fruit salad with frozen
        vanilla yoghurt 196
    raspberry jelly trifle 194
    red berry compote with yoghurt
        and honey 40
dips
    homous 218
    salsa cruda 217
    smoky chipotle 218
dressings
    honey and mustard 217
    soy and ginger 217
    yoghurt raita 217
    zingy salad 64
drinks
    Bellini cardinale 208, **209**
    home-made limeade 210, **211**
    The Homewood 214
    iced cardamom coffee 212, **213**
    peach mojito 206
    zinc bar punch 207
    see also smoothies

eggs
    poached egg with smoked trout
        on wholemeal toast 44
    window-garden herb omelette 46, **47**
Eton mess 198, **199**
exercise 14

feta cheese
    beetroot, mint and feta topping
        for jacket potato 170
    Greek salad 62, **63**

fish
    piquant marinade for 118
    fishcakes smoked haddock and
        parsley 154, **155**
    see also individual fish e.g. cod,
        salmon etc.
French onion soup 72, **73**
frittata
    spinach and cherry tomato 164
fruit 13 *see also* individual names
fruit salad
    marshmallow fruit salad with frozen
        vanilla yoghurt 196
fusilli con zucchini e pomodori 182, **183**

garlic
    gazpacho 81
    lemony-garlic crayfish and pea
        shoots on rye 54
gazpacho 81
ginger
    seared ginger and soy tuna with
        vegetable noodles 152
    soy and ginger dressing 217
goat's cheese
    baked goat's cheese and chicory
        salad 178, **179**
granola, crunchy 35, **34**
grapefruit juice
    The Homewood 214
Greek salad 62, **63**
gremolata, parsley 42

haddock
    smoked haddock and parsley
        fishcakes 154, **155**
halloumi and tomato kebabs 130
harissa-spiced chicken with bean
    and couscous salad 100, **101**
herbs
    window-garden herb omelette 46, **47**
Homewood, The 214
homous 218
honey
    and mustard dressing 217
    red berry compote with yoghurt
        and 40
horseradish
    rare beef with horseradish and
        watercress on wholemeal 54
hot-and-sour prawn noodle soup 86, **87**

iced cardamom coffee 212, **213**

jacket potatoes 168
    beetroot, mint and feta topping 170
    tricolore topping 170
    tuna, spring onions, lemon, pepper
        and capers topping 170
jerked chicken with fresh mango salsa 106
Jerusalem artichoke soup 85

kebabs
    halloumi and tomato 130
    lemony Greek lamb 130
    sticky lamb 126
kedgeree 45
kidney beans
    Texas chilli con carne 131
kiwi, banana and lime sunshine smoothie 36
koftas
    skinny lamb and spinach 119

labels, nutritional 14
lamb
    braised lamb shanks 132, **133**
    chops with a twist 120, **121**
    hotpot 110, **111**
    lemony Greek lamb kebabs 130
    skinny lamb and spinach koftas 119
    sticky lamb kebab 126
lasagne, seafood 140, **141**
lemons
    creamy lemon-coriander
        chicken curry with red peppers 96, **97**
    lamb chops with a twist 120,**121**
    lemony Greek lamb kebabs 130
    lemony-garlic crayfish and pea shoots
        on rye 54
    pork chops with lemon and sage 122,
        123
    preserved 55
    sardines with cucumber,
    lemon and flat-leaf parsley on toast 78
lentils
    dahl with okra and sweet potatoes 173
    hearty vegetable and lentil soup 74
    Puy lentils and coriander salad 65
limeade, home-made 210, **211**
linguine with sausage and cherry
        tomatoes 124, **125**

mangoes
    jerked chicken with fresh mango
        salsa 106
    prawn, avocado and mango wraps
        with coriander 60
maple syrup chicken 99, **98**
marinades 116
    beer marinade for steak 118
    piquant marinade for fish 118
    spicy marinade for chicken 118
marmite and avocado on toast 78
marshmallow fruit salad with frozen
        vanilla yoghurt 196
menu plans 18—25
Mexican turkey tacos 102
mint
    beetroot, mint and feta topping for
        jacket potato 170
    Vietnamese beef and mint salad 57, **56**
    yoghurt raita dressing 217
molasses
    wholewheat molasses muffins 41
mousse

dark chocolate and coffee 200, **201**
mozzarella cheese
    tricolore topping for jacket potato 170
muffins
    chocolate-banana sunflower 69, **68**
    wholewheat molasses 41
mushrooms
    beef shin and mushroom casserole 127
    chicken and mushroom curry 103
    chicken and mushroom risotto 104, **105**
    roast bacon, tomatoes and mushrooms
        with parsley gremolata 42, **43**
mussels 148, **149**
mustard
    honey and mustard dressing 217

noodles
    hot-and-sour prawn noodle soup 86, **87**
    seared ginger and soy tuna with
        vegetable 152
    spicy-sweet Thai 145

okra
    dahl with okra and sweet potato 173
omelette
    window-garden herb 46, **47**
onions
    French onion soup 72, **73**
    Panackelty 112
    pastry-free chive and onion quiche 172
    toad-in-the-hole with onion gravy 115,
        114
oranges
    spiced carrot and orange soup 84
orecchiette alla Pugliese 180
oriental tuna stir-fry 144

paella fried rice 153
pak choi
    seared ginger and soy tuna with
        vegetable noodles 152
Panackelty 112
pancakes
    coconut and banana 38, **39**
Parmesan
    roast asparagus on rocket with a
        Parmesan vinaigrette 176, **177**
parsley
    prawn and parsley couscous salad 55
    roast bacon, tomatoes and mushrooms
        with parsley gremolata 42, **43**
    sardines with cucumber, lemon and
        flat-leaf parsley on toast 78
    smoked haddock and parsley
        fishcakes 154, **155**
pasta
    cauliflower and pasta cheese bake 165
    fusilli con zucchini e pomodori 182,
        183
    linguine with sausage and cherry
        tomatoes 124, **125**
    orecchiette alla Pugliese 180
    seafood lasagne 140, **141**

spicy Italian coley 142, **143**
pastry-free chive and onion quiche 172
pea shoots
    lemony-garlic crayfish and pea
        shoots on rye 54
peaches
    Amaretto-amaretti 192, **193**
    mojito 206
peas
    Maltese pea and cumin soup 80
    stuffed butternut squash with sweet
        peppers 184, **185**
peppers
    creamy lemon-coriander chicken
        curry with red 96, **97**
    stuffed butternut squash with
        sweet 184, **185**
peppery hot-smoked salmon
    open sandwich on granary bread 54
poached egg with smoked trout on
    wholemeal toast 44
porchetta 130
pork
    chops with lemon and sage 122, **123**
    Normandy pork fillet 136, **137**
    porchetta 130
portion sizes 12
potatoes
    dahl with okra and sweet 173
    lamb hotpot 110, **111**
    panackelty 112
    spinach and cherry tomato frittata 164
    sweet potato and apple soup 79
    see also jacket potatoes
prawn(s)
    hot-and-sour prawn noodle soup 86, **87**
    paella fried rice 153
    and parsley couscous salad 55
    prawn, avocado and mango wraps
        with coriander 60
    seafood lasagne 140, **141**
    spicy-sweet Thai noodles 145
preserved lemons 55
prosciutto
    cod saltimbocca 146, **147**
Prosecco
    Bellini cardinale 208, **209**
Puy lentil and coriander salad 65

quiche
    garden-fresh 162, **163**
    pastry-free chive and onion 172

raspberries
    Bellini cardinale 208, **209**
    raspberry jelly trifle 194
ratatouille 184
ready-prepared food 15
red berry compote with yoghurt
    and honey 40
red peppers *see* peppers
rice
    broad bean and bacon risotto 113

cardamom-scented basmati 173
chicken and mushroom risotto 104,
    105
chickpea, spinach and cashew nut
    korma with pilaf 166, **167**
cooking perfect 93
kedgeree 45
oven-roasted ratatouille with brown
    rice 181
paella fried 153
Southern wild rice and Cajun
    chicken salad 61
toasted ground 56
tuna and brown rice salad 66
risotto
    broad bean and bacon 113
    chicken and mushroom 104, **105**
rocket
    roast asparagus on rocket with a
        Parmesan vinaigrette 176, **177**
rosemary
    sea bass fillets in a piquant tomato
        and rosemary sauce 159, **158**
rum
    peach mojito 206
    zinc bar punch 207

sage
    pork chops with lemon and 122, **123**
salads
    baked goat's cheese and chicory 178,
        179
    coleslaw 126
    Coronation chicken 67
    Greek 62, **63**
    harissa-spiced chicken with bean
        and couscous 100, **101**
    prawn and parsley couscous 55
    Puy lentil and coriander 65
    seared fresh tuna Niçoise 51, **50**
    Southern wild rice and Cajun
        chicken 61
    tuna and brown rice 66
    Vietnamese beef and mint 57, **56**
    warm chicken liver and apple 107
    see also dressings
salmon
    kedgeree 45
    peppery hot-smoked salmon open
        sandwich on granary bread 54
    seafood lasagne 140, **141**
    steam-cooked salmon with soy
        sauce 150, **151**
    see also smoked salmon
salsa
    cruda 217
    mango 106
sandwiches 52
    lemony-garlic crayfish and pea
        shoots on rye 54
    peppery hot-smoked salmon open
        sandwich on granary bread 54
    rare beef with horseradish and

watercress on wholemeal 54
sardines with cucumber, lemon and
    flat-leaf parsley on toast 78
sausages
    linguine with sausage and cherry
        tomatoes 124, **125**
    toad-in-the-hole with onion gravy
        115, **114**
sea bass fillets in a piquant tomato
    and rosemary sauce 159, **158**
seafood lasagne 140, **141**
seasoning, zesty 134
smoked haddock and parsley fishcakes
    154, **155**
smoked salmon
    wrap-around Manhattan 60
smoked trout
    poached egg with smoked trout
        on wholemeal toast 44
smoky chipotle dip 218
smoothies
    kiwi, banana and lime sunshine 36
    Mo'Bay 37
snacks 12
soups
    celeriac 85
    French onion 72, **73**
    gazpacho 81
    hearty vegetable and lentil 74
    hot-and-sour prawn noodle 86, **87**
    Jerusalem artichoke 85
    Maltese pea and cumin 80
    roast beetroot and apple 82, **83**
    spiced carrot and orange 84
    spicy Thai butternut squash 75
    sweet potato and apple 79
soy sauce
    seared ginger and soy tuna with
        vegetable noodles 152
    soy and ginger dressing 217
    steam-cooked salmon with 150, **151**
spinach
    and cherry tomato frittata 164
    chickpea, spinach and cashew nut
        korma with pilaf 166, **167**
    skinny lamb and spinach koftas 119
spring onions
    tuna, spring onions, lemon, pepper and
    capers toping for jacket potatoes 170
squash
    creamy chicken curry 94
    spicy Thai butternut squash soup 75
    stuffed butternut squash with sweet
        peppers 184, **185**
starchy foods 13
steam-cooked salmon with soy sauce
    150, **151**
stir fry
    five-spice chicken with a vegetable
        93, **92**
    oriental tuna 144
    sweet chilli tofu 171
strawberry(ies)

Bellini cardinale 208, **209**
Eton mess 198, **199**
Mo'Bay smoothie 37
sponge 202, **203**
stuffed butternut squash with sweet
    peppers 184, **185**
sunflower seeds
    chocolate-banana sunflower muffins
    69, **68**
sweet chilli tofu stir fry 171
sweet potato(es)
    and apple soup 79
    dahl with okra and 173

tacos
    Mexican turkey 102
tarragon chicken 95
tian
    Provencal vegetable 174, **175**
toad-in-the-hole with onion gravy 115, **114**
toast 76
    marmite and avocado on 78
    sardines with cucumber, lemon
        and flat-leaf parsley on 78
    tomato 78
toasted ground rice 56
tofu
    sweet chilli tofu stir fry 171
tomato(es)
    fusilli con zucchini e pomodori 182, **183**
    gazpacho 81
    Greek salad 62, **63**
    halloumi and tomato kebabs 130
    linguine with sausage and cherry 124,
        125
    roast bacon, tomatoes and mushrooms
        with parsley gremolata 42, **43**
    salsa cruda 217
    sea bass fillets in a piquant tomato
        and rosemary sauce 159, **158**
    spinach and cherry tomato frittata 164
    toast 78
    tricolore topping for jacket potato 170
trout
    English trout cooked in paper 156, **157**
    poached egg with smoked trout on
        wholemeal toast 44
tuna
    and brown rice salad 66
    oriental tuna stir-fry 144
    seared fresh tuna Niçoise 51, **50**
    seared ginger and soy tuna with
        vegetable noodles 152
    tuna, spring onions, lemon, pepper and
        capers topping for jacket potato 170
turkey
    club wrap 60
    Mexican turkey tacos 102

vegetables 13
    five-spice chicken with a vegetable
        stir-fry 93, **92**
    hearty vegetable and lentil soup 74

oriental tuna stir-fry 144
oven-roasted ratatouille with brown
    rice 181
Provencal vegetable tian 174, **175**
sweet chilli tofu stir fry 171
Vietnamese beef and mint salad 57, **56**

warm chicken liver and apple salad 107
watercress
    rare beef with horseradish and
        watercress on wholemeal 54
wholewheat molasses muffins 41
wraps 58
    club 60
    prawn, avocado and mango wraps
        with coriander 60
    wrap-around Manhattan 60

yoghurt
    Eton mess 198, **199**
    kiwi, banana and lime sunshine
        smoothie 36
    marshmallow fruit salad with frozen
        vanilla 196
    Mo'Bay smoothie 37
    raita dressing 217
    red berry compote with yoghurt
        and honey 40

zinc bar punch 207
zingy salad 64

Recipe acknowledgements

Crunchy granola Frances Thorne
Coconut and banana pancakes Holly Brenchley
Chocolate-banana sunflower muffins Michelle Nelson
Banana loaf Laura Alden
Hearty vegetable and lentil soup Emma Ross
Spicy Thai butternut squash soup Lisa Simon
French onion soup Trish Colvill
Sweet potato and apple soup Sarah Herschy
Hot-and-sour prawn noodle soup Holly Brenchley
Harissa-spiced chicken with bean and couscous salad
Rachel Derrick
Maple syrup chicken Sarah Herschy
Creamy chicken curry Jane Cooper
Five-spice chicken with a vegetable stir-fry Lucy Moore
Chicken and mushroom risotto Jessica Bogris
Mexican turkey tacos Sarah Herschy
Panackelty Jane Cooper
Lamb hotpot Lisa Jackson
Broad bean and bacon risotto Emma Gillaspy
Tasty toad-in-the-hole with onion gravy Emma Ross
Spicy Italian coley Emma Hills
Steam-cooked salmon with soy sauce Nilu Prentis
Seafood lasagne Laura Alden
Oriental tuna stir-fry Adriane Green
Spicy-sweet Thai noodles Katherine Knight
Seared ginger and soy tuna with vegetable noodles
Holly Brenchley
Paella fried rice Holly Brenchley

Luxury cauliflower and pasta cheese bake
Holly Brenchley
Chickpea, spinach and cashew nut korma with pilaf
Peter Russell
Garden-fresh quiche Catheryn Kilgarriff
Spinach and cherry tomato frittata Cherie Goold
Raspberry jelly trifle Laura Bond
Guiltlessly delicious fudge brownies Pamela Meliza
Amaretto-amaretti peaches Vivienne Cudd
Couscous cake Claire White
Marshmallow fruit salad with frozen vanilla yoghurt
Katrina Franken
Eton mess Jane Cooper
Peach mojito Holly Brenchley
Zingy salad Jane Cooper
Tuna and brown rice salad Jane Cooper
Coronation chicken salad Jessica Bogris
Tarragon chicken Rosemary Gardener
Creamy lemon-coriander chicken curry with
red peppers Becca Paterson
Chicken and mushroom curry Jane Darbey
Skinny lamb and spinach koftas Trish Colvill
Sticky lamb kebab Lisa Jackson
Beef shin and mushroom casserole Jane Cooper
Sweet chilli tofu stir-fry Kelly Louise Simons
Chocolate crispy cakes Jessica Gray
Light strawberry sponge Katherine Christensen

Kay Plunkett-Hogge

Kay Plunkett-Hogge was born in Bangkok, Thailand and spent many years working in film and fashion in London, New York, Bangkok and Los Angeles until finally she decided to follow her true passion – food. In addition to cooking for private clients, Kay works as a food writer, stylist and presenter, and launched her popular food blog, A Terribly Greedy Girl, in 2007. She runs a bespoke catering company, Kay Cooks For You, and teaches one-on-one cookery classes, as well as taking small groups of foodies on exclusive Food Adventure trips twice a year. She lives in south west London with her husband and a pair of crazy cats, and is a keen balcony kitchen gardener.

Acknowledgements

Tiger Aspect Productions would like to extend a big thank you to all of the cookyourselfthin.co.uk users who entered the competition and let us share your stories. Without you this book would not have been possible. And thanks too to everyone at Weight Loss Resources for introducing us all. At Penguin it's been great to work once more with such a committed team, particularly Kate Adams and Sarah Rollason. As ever, we are immensely grateful for the participation of Gordon Wise at Curtis Brown and Jo McGrath, Jamie Munro, Jenny Spearing and Elaine Foster at Tiger Aspect. And finally, a huge thanks to Kay Halsey, Lynne Garton, Kay Plunkett-Hogge and Trish Davies who, together with our wonderful competition winners, have produced a fabulous book.

Cook Yourself Thin Online

You too can cook yourself thin with these specially developed tools to help you eat well and lose weight:

Track calories and see how many you have used up in each meal and how many you have left for the day

See the proportion of fat, protein and carbs in your food, and how many grams of fibre – giving you the control to balance your diet

Keep notes about food and drink for the day, how you felt and what affected what you ate and drank

Search for recipes by calorie content or your favourite ingredients, or browse through the recipe categories for inspiration

Create and calorie-count your own recipes, and see what difference it makes to the calories when you change quantities or swap ingredients, helping you drop the pounds without dropping your favourite dishes

Add recipes to your Diary, from the database or from the list of recipes you have created

Set a weight loss goal; see how many calories you need to get there and the date you can expect to reach your goal

Speed up or slow down your rate of loss depending on what suits you at the time. You can even go onto 'maintenance calories' for times when you need to relax but don't want to put weight on. Great for holidays and Christmas

Track your measurements and view your weight graph – there's nothing more motivating than a nice downward line!

Get support – whatever you're going through, the chances are that other members can relate to it. They understand exactly what you mean because they've been there themselves

Get ideas and inspiration – real life practical answers to situations you face from ''What shall I have for lunch?'' to ''How do I cope with evening munchies?''

Add the IDs of your buddies to your friends list and you can see when they're online

Start cooking yourself thin today! Join from as little as £7.50 a month

www.cookyourselfthin.co.uk